OLD AND SMART

To Collette

Betty Heckenson

OLD AND SMART

WOMEN AND THE ADVENTURE OF AGING

Betty Nickerson

HARBOUR PUBLISHING

Madeira Park, British Columbia

HARBOUR PUBLISHING
P.O. Box 219
Madeira Park, BC Canada V0N 2H0

Page design by Gaye Hammond
Page composition by Vancouver Desktop Publishing Centre
Author photograph by Jennifer Modigliani

Printed and bound in Canada

To invite Betty Nickerson to speak, please contact:
    R.R. 3 Yellow Point Road
    Ladysmith, BC Canada V0R 2E0

Canadian Cataloguing in Publication Data

Nickerson, Betty, 1922-
   Old and smart

   Includes bibliographical references and index.
   ISBN 1-55017-120-8

   1. Aged women—Canada. 2. Aged women—United States.
I. Title.
HQ1061.N68 1995   305.26'0971   C95-910408-9

For my Age Mates

CONTENTS

Preface   9

CHAPTER 1
Don't Believe Anyone Under Sixty   19

CHAPTER 2
Someday I'll Find You   33

CHAPTER 3
Our Life   38
Our Alphabet of Time   65

CHAPTER 4
People with the Most Birthdays Live Longest   67

CHAPTER 5
The Way We Are   73
Affirmations of Maturity   88

CHAPTER 6
Getting Clear   89

CHAPTER 7
I'm Just a Housewife   99

CHAPTER 8
The Healing Mind   111

CHAPTER 9
The Care and Treatment of Doctors   137

CHAPTER 10
Good Medicine   158

CHAPTER 11
Walk to the Fountain of Youth   178

CHAPTER 12
Give Us This Day Our Daily Bread   184

CHAPTER 13
The Memory of . . .   195

CHAPTER 14
The Adventure of Sex   206

CHAPTER 15
Loose Threads   227

CHAPTER 16
Ways and Means   249
100 Things To Do that Don't Cost Any Money   270

CHAPTER 17
Bridging Troubled Waters   272

CHAPTER 18
Go Softly Into That Bright Light   289

CHAPTER 19
Follow Your Bliss   305

Acknowledgments   315

Sources of Interest   317

Index   323

PREFACE

B ooks are like tapestries. They are made from hundreds of threads woven into meaningful patterns. The object of art is to create order out of chaos, and to keep in mind appropriateness and usefulness, always alert to beauty. We weave our life's tapestry with threads of observation, imagination and opportunity textured with love.

We each work at our own looms warped with cords of time, weft with a never-ending flow of change, and thus create the matrix of each individual life. I perceive my loom, sturdy and wide, placed firmly upon the Earth, woven with the colors of my years. Half of my life was spent in the United States, the second half in Canada, living in cities, small towns and rural areas. The design evolves continuously. The background is woven with quite ordinary shades of beige and brown with touches of gold among inevitable grays. Here and there it is shot with clear colors of great brilliance—ideas, dreams, discoveries, friends, sorrows, births, deaths and joy—moments lived, invested with spirit and love.

Some weavers set out to make definite patterns with clearly marked edges. I have never been that certain about my design, nor, I'm finally able to admit, do I wish to be. There is so much to discover, take in, choose, and try in the changing picture of our

9

lives. If the weaver "goes with the flow" as our flower children told us, unexpected textures appear. One may discover new colors, find opportunities to exchange threads with others, or learn to spin for oneself.

Eventually, as tapestry or book comes together, the pattern takes shape. It is not what I thought it would be in the beginning. The pattern, like life itself, is always becoming. It changes with the passage of my days through time. I thought the pattern would be complete now that my loom is at least three-quarters full, but I find there are choices still to be made. I have both the desire and the opportunity to enhance the colors of the sky.

Assuming you are a woman who has seen fifty to eighty summers and looked upon the full moon eight hundred times or more, the broad events of your life will be similar to mine. We have lived in dramatic times. During our lives, the world has undergone the most extensive changes of any period in history. We have witnessed extraordinary transformation at every level. "Progress" has altered our lives dramatically: changes in family structure, scientific discoveries, medical advances, extended life expectancy, global communication, transportation, energy, wars, and the invention of ever more terrible weapons designed to lay waste to whole populations. We ageful North American women have lived through deep Depression into the most affluent period in history.

Our affluence has not been without consequences. Nature herself has been changed. While life has been extended and enhanced for many of the world's people, children still die of hunger. The cost of our enhancement is not yet truly understood. Many of the great achievements are very dangerous, and we have no idea where to put the garbage. When we raised questions about what was happening, we were politely assured that it has all been for development and the good of mankind. We naively imagined that included us. We women of age have served as wives and mothers to the men who engineered the changes. I wonder, could we not have been more vigilant? Can we now help the planet and our multitudes step back from the brink of chaos?

We approach our sixth, seventh, eighth decades to find ourselves at a moment of in-between. We are poised amid a half-remembered past, time-swept into an often frightening tomorrow with few guideposts for the many years ahead of us. There are times when I feel infirm, more times when the world seems infirm around me. Like you, I have survived war, Depression, disease, childbirth and astonishing technological changes. It isn't over yet. In recent years I have begun to carry a deep, abiding sorrow for the state of our Earth and her threatened creatures—the Earth whose riches once seemed infinite now appears to be compromised on numerous fronts.

As I write this I am seventy-two years old. In childhood I walked alone and unafraid through town and forest, ate berries and shoots of wild asparagus from the side of the road. I drank from creeks that ran beside the farmer's field, swam in rivers, bathed carefree in a warming sun. Today, I must warn my granddaughters against such delights!

I emerged from the certainties of a small Oregon town into great cities and an ever-widening vista of a planet with interdependent living things, a planet now known to be at risk—a cherished blue spot in an expanding universe, for we have seen our planet photographed from outer space. Unprecedented millions of women are in the same time frame with us, preparing, in due course, to experience The Mystery which is greater than all the others and which comes eventually to every living thing.

It is astonishing to realize we have traveled so far in time only to discover that few knew we were coming. Society and governments seem surprised to find millions of older women appearing at this time in history. Since we are virtually unknown for who we are, what we care about and what we can do, we must speak for ourselves. Society's attitude toward age and aging urgently needs readjustment. We are entitled to an honest representation of the potential and vitality of today's mature women, far different from the absurd stereotypes by which we are often portrayed.

Much waits to be discovered, comprehended and applied if we are to truly understand the possibilities of our mature years. Our challenge is to write ourselves into existence, make the truth real to ourselves and others. For the sake of our daughters and generations of females still unborn, we have an assignment to clarify women's role in society and inscribe the possibilities of age on the guideposts to the future. By our very invisibility we are free to create our image, establish our rules, decide what we wish to do with our lives, and *do* it.

We North American women have attained the long life for which generations before us have wished. We are pioneers in a new age that has much need of common sense and even greater need of wisdom. We are foremothers of millions of older women who will appear as our "baby boom" daughters age. What we create in our maturity will be our gift to them.

This book has little to say about averages, statistics or double-blind experiments. It cannot be considered a scientific research project. Instead of a systematic counting of things or people, I've tried to listen beyond the numbers to the *sense* of the many women I've met. Certainly statistics have their uses but they are cold and impersonal. Numbers cannot describe the raw courage of the woman now in her seventies who told me about her "dust bowl" experiences. Numbers cannot capture the joy of a ninety-year-old immigrant woman seeing her great-granddaughter deliver the commencement address in a language barely understood, nor the triumph of the woman who took me to a hillside to see "her" forest nursed into being from tiny seedlings planted half a century ago.

No dollars-and-cents account does justice to the ingenuity with which the majority of older women manage their affairs. Despite years and years of contributions to the well-being of community and nation—bearing and raising children, creating homes for families, providing back-up for husbands, spending time in the

12

workplace—older women are disproportionately found on the bottom rung of the financial ladder. Many of us live below the poverty line but manage finances with a genius that would earn distinction in the board rooms of the nation. We teem with inventiveness. We cope!

The ideas and opinions included here are my synthesis of the thoughts and experiences of hundreds of women. I have talked informally with my Age Mates wherever we met. It's been enjoyable. Insights and bits of information have come through casual conversations in all sorts of places—at bus stops, in shopping centers, at checkout counters, bank lineups, bookstores and doctors' offices, and while the pharmacist types out the inevitable prescription. We've talked before and after meetings, at the hairdresser's, the unemployment centre, the post office, the laundromat, on trains, planes and city buses. We have spoken with one another at weddings, celebrations, protest demonstrations and my sister's funeral. We have talked about the matters which brought us together, our concerns of the moment, our expectations of tomorrow.

We've spoken of sorrow and joy, about the cost of living, the environment, endangered species, gardens, pets and house plants, changing lives and changing times, the health of the world, and about that delightful bonus of aging, grandchildren. I have found us committed to our own future and the future which will continue through our grandchildren. We worry about what will be left to assure quality for their lifetimes and the planet's.

More conversations took place in study groups, during retreats, after meditation sessions, at pot luck dinners, in parks, at auctions, during ballet rehearsals and theater intermissions, and once at a bingo parlor. I've found friends in strangers at pottery classes, during walks along the beach and through the forest, at soup kitchens, day care centers, political rallies and Peace Walks in several cities.

Since the publication of an earlier, self-published version of *Old and Smart*, I have met hundreds more women through the mail, and my life has been enriched by your letters and comments.

Women have told me how *Old and Smart* has amused and reinforced them in their search for more dynamic aging. Lots of fears about growing "old" have dissipated. Women are discovering new possibilities, seeing new vistas open before them and finding other ageful women with whom to share the adventure of aging. They have sought to "follow their bliss," to gather a new sense of self in their maturity. The letters signal a powerful wave of consciousness developing among women in all walks of life and of various ages.

Some women have written inspiring accounts of experiences from "olden" days, others write about problems they face now and enlightening insights about enduring life's tragedies and celebrating life's joys. They are a profound demonstration of the power of women and the remarkable strengths among us. My belief that the true history of cultures resides in the experience and wisdom of women is greatly reinforced.

From a Portland social worker: "This book has been needed for years. I'm glad you wrote it." From Seattle: "I feel I am a better person from reading your book, certainly I feel better about growing old. I'm 87." "I know the rest of my life can be full of adventure. I'm finally letting myself appreciate who I am"—from a new friend in Thunder Bay. From Toronto: "Your talk about Mother Earth made me stop and listen to the world around me." From Detroit: "For the first time since I was a girl I stood and listened to nature. It brought great tears of joy, returning to a long forgotten place."

"I laughed or amen-ed on every page." "Send two more copies; I'm aging rapidly." And from a seventeen-year-old, "I gave my mother a copy for Christmas, she gave it to my grandmother, and my grandmother insisted that *I* read it, then we all went to Scotland." Another reader advised, "You left out something important in the list of 100 Things to Do. Procrastinate. It's easy, doesn't cost anything, and you can do it forever." Actually, I thought about that. I even got a book on procrastination, but I haven't read it yet. Thanks anyway.

Some letters brought me to tears: "My dearest friend is dying from terminal brain cancer. I visit her every night to read a few pages from *Old and Smart*. It helps her laugh. I'm saving the beautiful chapter on your Near Death Experience to read on the last day of her life." Another time in Toronto a beautiful, tiny woman wept her story on my shoulder, telling me this was the first time she had ventured away from home since her husband died six months before. "I'm so glad I came to hear you. Maybe I can feel like a human being again after all."

Quite a number of you picked up on the picture of my cat, Pitzi. She even gets fan letters! "Dear Pitzi, My mother has been much happier since she read your mother's book!"—signed by Muffin with a big fuzzy paw. Now I have *cats*. A delightful, rambunctious orange creature scrambled out of the sea, and has complicated our lives ever since. She was so brave and wanted to live so much that we fed her, washed her off, took her to the vet and called her . . . *Magnificat*. Thank you for the cat pictures, postcards, letterheads and paw prints.

Along with the thick file of correspondence, I've been invited to speak to groups of women, large and small, as well as on numerous radio and television programs. Sometimes I walk into a room of a hundred or more smiling women, a third to half of them wearing something purple. It's a wonderful sight. Purple has become the badge of Age Mates.

By far the most frequent comment was to say that we Age Mates need to find a way to get together, a chance to share our experiences and support one another in this unscripted adventure into age. There is a great desire to establish guideposts to live by, role models to emulate and respect. Which, of course, is something we do for each other simply because we know more about the lives of older women than anyone else.

These many comments and a very real dream, resulted in the first gathering of Amazing Grays in October 1993, in Parksville, BC. There, for one remarkable weekend, women celebrated together, created a rite of passage into our cronehood, enjoyed each other's company, exercised our creativity, laughed and sang together and saw new paths before us.

We weren't all "Grays" but we were all amazing. About a quarter of the women were considerably younger. We gave them the special designation of AGIT, Amazing Grays in Training, and they enjoyed it as much as anyone. Since that time the idea has spread to other communities and it appears that gatherings of Amazing Grays are becoming widely shared events. In the United States women gather as members of the Crone Counsel. We could all facilitate such events. All it takes is a venue and an extrovert.

We were so inspired by that first gathering that we decided to do it again in October 1994. There was so much joy. Within a circle of 167 women in a wonderful, candlelit room filled with drum beats tuned to our hearts, each woman who wanted to claim her crone-hood was presented with a certificate reading:

> Welcome to the Sisterhood of Crones
> Welcome to the honor only Time bestows
>> Stand firmly on our good green Earth;
>> Love her as Mother who nurtures all.
>> Speak the Wisdom of your years;
>> Enhance the Good as you know it.
>> Offer guidance from experience.
>> Live lightly on the Earth;
>> Raise your spirits to the sky.
>> Wear your Crown of Time with pride,
>>> with Joy, and Love.
> These years will manifest the best
>> you have been and all you will become.
>> Welcome
> Take your place in the Sisterhood of Crones
>> Blessed Be

Among many wise women whose works I consulted, I wish especially to thank the late Dr. Marion Hilliard, who wrote her special book, *A Woman Doctor Looks at Love and Life*, nearly half a century ago. Rereading it after all those years—after woman's lib, after the Charter of Rights in Canada, the Equal Rights Amendment in the United States, after the rise of the new feminism—I was convinced that the only way I could write honestly about the lives of women was by using the first person. Coming to terms with myself in the written word has been difficult. The effort has significantly changed the composition of my "tapestry."

I sincerely thank the many women who have contributed their personal experiences and viewpoints to this collective account of aging in North America. It is a joyful tale! Much more can be written. Thank you for all your kind words, your books and stories, hundreds of cat pictures, the laughter and tears, but most of all for the inspiration you have been.

By sheer weight of numbers we are a significant factor in the unfolding of our culture and our world. The experiences we have acquired from decades of nurturing is urgently needed in the greater society. Even more important is our experience in resolving conflicts. When we look back on our years of mothering, and the unending task of settling conflicts within family and community, we will realize how valuable our experiences have been, and how desperately they are needed on the world stage. Competitive cultures wither and die amid great chaos; co-operative cultures flower.

You may find yourself here as part of this amazing sisterhood.

Rooms full of women have requested copies of the poem with which I end most of my talks. It defines our place in the cosmos.

To Thine Own Self Be True

We are Spirits wrapped in the stuff of the Earth.
Rivers of oceans flow in our veins,
Mountains of minerals build our bones.
Acres of growing things give us strength and sinew
We fill our lungs with the breath of trees.
For we are of the Earth, and the Earth is in us
Making us holy. Honor Her whole.

—Betty Nickerson
February 1995

CHAPTER 1

DON'T BELIEVE
ANYONE UNDER SIXTY

*I wonder if there's time to do
half the things I've wanted to?*
—Age Mate, 75

The culture of North America surrounds old age with myth. These myths include little about the positive side of aging. We are exposed to a seemingly endless list of problems, illnesses and infirmities said to be a true account of age. We have to learn for ourselves that we may be old, but we are also smart. Although our hearts sometimes fill with bittersweet memories of youth, very, very few women would willingly return to the anguish of immaturity.

My first indication that *old* had actually arrived came from the income tax form. There's a line somewhere that entitles the claimant to deduct a bunch of money. Anytime the government allows ordinary people to keep tax money indicates a special occasion!

Year by year the time to deduct those extra dollars crept up. I noted it casually. 1916. Oh yeah, that's the year So-and-so was born. 1918. That was the year World War One ended. Then it was 1920. 1921 showed up, and I thought to myself, getting close! Then, Bingo! 1922! That was it! What a shock! My birth year! I didn't know whether to rejoice over the deduction, or grow melancholy at the number. It was the coming of Age! It meant I was, horror of horrors, officially, irrevocably, governmentally *old*.

How could it be? I didn't *feel* old. I had never felt better. Life seemed *far* from over. Except as an abstract idea, I hadn't noticed many changes as the years piled up. However, the youthfulness of doctors, teachers, and brides *was* noticeable. But there was Time, measured tax return after tax return and suddenly, it was my turn. It just sort of happened.

With the exception of the fuss made by people approaching forty, I didn't find any who thought of *themselves* as old. Old is somewhere down the line. Most women I asked said they thought they might be old in about ten years.

I've been enjoying that tax break for seven years! Being seventy-two is a bit of a shock, but also an acceptable excuse for doing what I've always wanted to do. My body is now my own. I'm free from childbearing, free from cramps and hot flashes, free from the lure of merchandised unreality, free from the phoneyness women often think they must endure. At long last I can be myself and I'm enjoying it more and more.

Our society does quite a lot to make this possible. Every month two checks arrive, one the standard Old Age Pension, the other a smaller one which accounts for the few years I was employed for minimal wages outside the home. They don't add up to a huge sum, but it is enough to live on—carefully. We women receive old age pension checks in our own right. For quite a few of our generation this is the first time we have had money in our own names.

> I'm going to spend my first pension check celebrating
> because I won't be around to spend the last one!
>
> —Age Mate, 65

The greater society wraps us about in special privileges. "Golden Agers" get reductions on train fares (assuming you can still find a train.) Where I live in British Columbia, "seniors" ride free on the ferries Monday through Thursday. If you pick the time right there are seniors' rates for theaters, concerts and swimming pools. Some restaurants, bakeries, drug stores, and service people extend special discounts. Most banks remove or reduce service charges. But be sure to ask. The kindness society displays to "seniors" is helpful, practical, much appreciated, and completely impersonal.

I take advantage of all these privileges. Sage age saves! Not everyone feels that way apparently. I've been told that some people, mainly men, refuse reductions even though they are obviously eligible. "They don't want anyone to think they are old," a waiter told me. "We no longer ask passengers if they wish free passage. You never can tell when they are going to throw a fit," a ferry purser said.

To insist on playing the charade of over-long youth is lonely, expensive, time-consuming and false. Yearning for youth is a kind of self-made handicap that holds us back, keeps us from discoveries that are ours to make. It takes too much time and energy to create a shell impermeable enough to camouflage one's nonrenewable natural resources. Staying artificially young can absorb all one's creativity. As one grows toward self-acceptance, the make-believe doesn't seem worth the struggle. It is more fun to explore this new territory, to make responsible, adventurous use of undiscovered wealth waiting to be revealed.

Sixty-five, seventy-two or any of those big numbers were unimaginable when we were young. Now it is ours! This is the "many happy returns of the day" wished at birthday parties! We have acquired the experience of time. We are here because we are supposed to be. Each of us is, as that wonderful essay "Desiderata" says, "a child of the Universe, no less than the trees and the stars."

There is no alternative to aging. It comes with being alive.

Besides, everybody's doing it! Age hang-ups, those devious little tricks some women (and quite a few men) play on others, or on themselves, are rather sad. The facts of age are established in many kinds of numbers—driver's licenses, marriage certificates, tax returns, all the paper society holds on us. It is just a number, and numbers neither define nor describe a human person.

So what do we do when we are technically "old"? There are few role models of healthy, capable women over sixty. The stereotype has us all in rocking chairs, snowy hair tied in buns, wearing aprons and being forever agreeable. Nonsense! I don't even own an apron, and I'm not always agreeable. These are images from an earlier time, perpetuated in the simple minds of advertisers who can't see what they are looking at.

We are what old age *is*! We have the exciting possibility of redefining age, creating the new paradigm, a new definition of age sorely needed in our society. If we do it well, our patterns will inspire generations who follow. For the moment our task is to figure out the best that aging can be, and go for it. We may indeed sit in rocking chairs and contemplate the miracles around us, *if we choose to do so.*

The conventional wisdom, derived mainly from "experts" who have not experienced age, is filled with prophesies of misery and general ignorance about the natural life processes known as aging. Outsiders seldom see the peace and contentment widely reported by women as they grow older. We must discover that information for ourselves. If we are going to be *old* women, let us create the best old age we can, and enjoy it. Rather than being diminished by age, women who believe in themselves are enhanced by the sum of their years. We are repositories of the experience and wisdom of our time. We need not be victimized by notions of decrepitude. We are Elders.

The four things society seems unable to understand about us are:
• We are self-reliant 95 percent of the time.

- We are not mere consumers to be seduced in the marketplace.
- We do not generally feel obliged to conduct ourselves as sex objects.
- We have at last the power to say "no!" and mean it.

Ageism, specifically as applied to older women, is possibly the last prejudice society openly permits. Ageism is not politically correct! Where newspapers, magazines and television would not risk referring to blacks, Jews, Hispanics, and increasingly, gays, there are no restrictions on making fun of "little old ladies." It perpetuates images that in no way resemble us, ascribes to us attitudes we do not hold, behavior we do not affect.

I have been wading through murky waters trying to learn the truth about growing old. There is something disturbing about a learned forty-year-old telling us about age. It is rather like the self-righteous ten-year-old insisting we shouldn't smoke, even if he's right. I find almost nothing written or said about being old to be true. To the best of my ability, I will speak the truth about my age and the discoveries I am making. Every woman has her own truth. For me, this is the best age so far and I am only beginning to understand its potential, no matter what others have to say about it. May you celebrate a similar truth.

Many women I've talked with express the feeling that their lives now are unimportant, that they lose in value as they grow older. To gain a better sense of women's worth we must ask some questions.

Why are we excluded from the accounts of our times?

Why is there so little recognition of the value of women's lives?

Why is the work produced by women's endless energy ignored?

Why is there so little mention of the care and nurture, the healing and the love we have given?

Why are we less than equal?

We must answer with a few questions of our own. Who preserved the harvest against the bitterness of winter? Who planted the gardens, ground the flour, raised the animals, spun the wool, wove the fabrics, dressed the skins, and welcomed the hunters home? Who brought new lives into the world? And who laid out the dead when life's work was over? Is it not possible that all human persons would feel more secure if they remembered that this dependable, nurturing energy has allowed civilization to endure? That same energy continues to serve, remaining separate from the politician's bottom line or the warrior's body count.

Woman's truth may not parallel historical records but history is written mainly by those who hold the power, by the "winners" in the violent struggle from the cave to the spaceship. Small notice is given to those who have loved and nourished—or the warriors who lost. Hold on to the truth of your life. It has validity and beauty.

Women have made formidable contributions in the fields of science, medicine, law, business and the arts. We have always been half or more of the population, but since women aren't making war, oppressing indigenous people or writing constitutions, we scarcely exist in official history. Surely there was more to women's part in the American Revolution than Betsy Ross snipping out stars with a single cut. This gifted designer was probably frustrated out of her mind with a burning desire to contribute to the dramatic events around her. In the war books of Canadian history the main contribution from women was young Laura Secord's decision to walk her cow through enemy lines, and claim to be lost. This courageous, nonviolent act proved more effective than muskets and so midwifed the infant that would be Canada.

Women suffer the fears and deprivation of war, not the spectacular sideshows. Although it may be grand sport for men of power, war is never fun for women. Throughout the struggles we bear our children, heal the sick and wounded, nurture the new generation. The history of woman is life-giving—to plant, reap and preserve, to spin, weave and sew, and to defend the home base.

So where were we? Since the population continued to grow,

women had to be *somewhere*. We know that numbers of *Filles de Roi* ("daughters of the king") were imported to Canada from among the poor women of France, but once chosen by trappers, they largely vanished from the record. Similarly, boatloads of English women faded into the forests to occupy log cabins they helped to build deep in the wilderness. Even the affluent few settled anonymously in their drawing rooms, embroidery hoops at the ready. All women were denied the vote for generations, classed with idiots and the criminally insane well into the nineteen hundreds. The right to be considered as "persons" equal before the law was won in *our* generation.

Women made it into print protesting slavery and again during the suffrage movement, remarked more for extremes of civil disobedience than for the quality of their ideas. Women were not trusted in the affairs of state, nor allowed to contribute directly to the great movements of the time. We were sometimes able to gain an audience for our views in the intimacy of pillow talk or drawing room conversations.

Women's social concerns are still discounted. We are often accused of being too emotional. This is a prime example of the double standard applied to human relations. Hate is also an emotion, ignited and perpetuated by men at war. The deadly sin of manly greed, the arrogance of manly power—all strong emotions! Why then do women's emotions of love, peace and equality disqualify us? Of course we are emotional! Acting with the heart not the fists, protecting our children, creating the nurturing ambience of homes, maintaining a base from which the men could go out to conquer and exploit, awaiting their safe return, accepting them in our beds, sheltering them from their wars and travels with woman's love—all this requires us to be emotional. These services are not cultivated through cold-blooded reason. Without women's labors, settlements do not come into being. The presence of women allows roots to grow, gives permanence to communities. The whole of North America might still be filled with rowdy trappers living it up in trading posts had we not come to share the work of nation-building.

If the real work of women is generally ignored in history, the role of older women is nowhere to be found. And we probably won't exist so long as we permit our grandchildren to be taught from the chronicles of conquest currently accepted as history.

Age is an opportunity to re-evaluate ourselves, to separate the worthwhile from the junk, weave new themes into our life stories, appreciate what we know and pass it on to those who wish to listen. Our experience is more practical than theoretical. Think how much useful information Depression-reared women have to share with today's young people eager to learn about recycling, reusing, remaking, renewal and that ancient art of mending. We have practical experience in self-sufficiency. What we know about the real cost of the wars we have witnessed will help reinforce the peace marchers.

We have lived with monumental changes in our sixty-plus years, many remarkable and inspiring, others life-and planet-threatening. We have coped and survived. Age gives us time to savor life's wonders, to combine experience and knowledge and help create a wiser world—a world which must eventually include women's values if it is to survive.

It is not my intention to be bitter about these oversights, but to add some sense of who *we* are to the record book. When we and others learn the truth about the essential contribution feminine characteristics make to the development of civilization, and have made throughout the ages, our self-esteem—and everyone else's—will benefit.

Older women are not alone in the quest to understand and grow. Younger women too pore over books, how-to articles, and research studies, desperately hoping to defeat Time, afraid to discover what lies beyond their trim figures and the rat race. Many prefer pain and deception rather than accepting the inevitable passage of time. We have been oversold on glorious youth, to the point where many refuse to accept maturity. Youth is a fashionable gown of great beauty, delightful when worn for the right occasions, but unbecoming at inappropriate times. There are new gowns for us, cloaks in wonderful colors with intriguing textures, found along fascinating avenues which only mature women may travel.

A new and different concept of aging will develop as we find our wings and recognize our strength. We are, after all, the fastest-growing section of the population, and we are smart. Collectively we have had the benefits of better nutrition, extraordinary innovations in health care, better living conditions and better education than any previous generation. We live longer, have traveled further and are generally more active than our grandmothers. Most aging women are eager to get on with their lives, to live fully and well. Even the helping professions are slowly shifting their focus from degeneration to life-enhancing potential.

There are millions of educated, healthy, experienced women of mature years in North America. Our talents combined with the cultural experiences of women everywhere give us a wealth of information from which to develop the best possible lives for ourselves, and forge new trails for our descendants. As in ancient times, women's culture is built cooperatively. We are free to focus on the best qualities of all the cultures, weaving them together to create a shining memorial to the strength of women.

As soon as we are willing to come to terms with the idea of age, we can choose what kind of *old* we will be. The prospects are limitless. Anything that can be imagined can come to pass, so ask your innermost self just what sort of person you would like to be, and make it so. It brings to mind the slogan of our hippie kids, "Be here now." Being is never a static position, but a dynamic direction toward an inexhaustible variety of possibilities waiting to be discovered both within and without. Dare to honor the need for spirituality born of love, not dogma.

Far from life being finished, getting old is a chance to start over. We have a good idea where mistakes were made, *and* where the flowers bloom. Individually and collectively we have wisdom and millions of bits of experience. How can we most creatively combine those bits to make the best possible intellectual, physical, social, economic space we can visualize? We can free ourselves from fads and false goals. Cut loose from the fetish of consumerism, learn to live more simply, demand less of Earth's finite resources, receive more from the true wealth which is the birthright of all living things and adopt life-based pursuits, the pursuits that lead not to profits or success, but to the creation of cultural riches. My guess is that by the time the baby boom generation reaches sixty, it will be fashionable to be old and living more in harmony with the planet.

> You can't have everything. Where would you put it?
> —Age Mate, 65

The majority of mature North American women have acquired most of the *things* they need. The desire for fast cars and fur coats has generally faded into wistfulness. Most of us have observed that *lots* of something, be it money or beauty or fame, doesn't assure contentment. Excess is immature. Whatever can one do with so much stuff? Some of it is valuable in monetary terms; more of it holds little measurable value, but is treasured as memories. Personally, I have no idea of what to do with accumulated things. I'd like to find a way to endow friends or institutions with appropriate items of special value, to give them away where the stories they tell will be appreciated. I would rather simplify my life than polish silver teapots.

How to simplify is another matter. Who, for example, would most appreciate an exquisitely decorated, ivory inlaid, unplayed sitar? Or my pioneer great-grandmother's hand-carved bowl in which she made butter for half a century? However much time we have left, let it be quality time, something more than counting, comparing, or dusting all those things!

One Age Mate of ninety-plus tried an interesting approach. She tactfully returned special gifts to the donors, saying she knew they had chosen things they themselves admired, and because of their good taste, she wanted them to have the pleasure of these special things now that she wouldn't be using them any longer.

That Age Mate happened to be my mother, and after the initial shock which quivered on the edge of rejection, I thought it a super idea. I greatly enjoy having the beautifully woven basket I lugged home from India, and my granddaughters shared a laugh with me over the piece of carnival glass purchased for a hard-earned quarter back in the thirties. They can't decide which of them should inherit it.

As we grow older we live in a different kind of economy, where less is more, where natural is naturally best, where the clutter of many acquisitions becomes only clutter. Part of the wisdom of a woman's age is to understand the meaning of enough. What seems most satisfying to me now is feeling whole, being at peace inside myself. I've been many places, seen many wonders, known tragedy, watched momentous events unfold, and sensed both anguish and excitement. I honestly don't want that sort of tension any longer.

My greatest joy is a dawning appreciation of my connection with the Earth. Life is enhanced through simple things like buds on trees, flowers in window boxes, a flight of birds, waves on the beach or across a field of ripening grain, the fragrance of wild roses, music, the sound of rain, the silence of snow, and most of all by five granddaughters and two extraordinary pussycats. There *is* a place for these things. Satisfactions, and there are many, now come from working with others sharing dreams of a better world, a cleaner environment, and making things.

In my travels from sea to sea in Canada, the United States and some forty-five other countries, I was so wrapped up in discovery and exploration that I scarcely noticed aging women until I became one of them. I couldn't relate to reference books filled with statistics measuring negative conditions. Besides, most of these were about old men. I didn't find myself in those pages. Of dozens of books and hundreds of articles, I found none written by an elderly woman who admitted it, or who wrote from that point of view. I have tried to do this. Now that I have reached life's transforming moment, I really *don't* trust anyone under sixty to describe me to myself. In the contest between experience and theory, experience carries the greater weight, experts to the contrary.

In the communications media of our times older women exist mainly as objects of parody and caricature. The stereotype of small, bent-over women with frizzy white hair, squeaky croaking voices, clumsy shoes and square-set hats bears little resemblance to the active, healthy women I know. In Canada, the outrageous and thoroughly delightful Raging Grannies use the media stereotype to make wonderful comic parody. Dressed in ridiculous combinations of out-dated fashions, the Raging Grannies sing about serious, topical events that reactionaries hate to hear. They say things the majority would hardly dare. And they leave everyone laughing.

We appear on television as the affluent "Golden Girls," which supplies a healthy dose of therapeutic laughter and shows us some great clothes. Older women may appear in commercials concerned with trivial matters, bent into uncommon shapes and speaking with distorted voices which advertisers apparently think will sell something. We are allowed to express delight when we get a telephone call from our grandchildren, but we are not to be seen speaking out about the kind of world they live in. Personally I resolve not to purchase any advertised products in which we appear as stupid, malleable old bats. If the advertisers' assessment of the audience is that inaccurate, their product must also be useless.

Those who wish to communicate with older women need to learn that we are different from men. We don't need macho. Few of the women I've known in my lifetime have devoted their lives to proving themselves in epic battles to subdue nature, catch the biggest fish, get the most money or acquire the most power. We don't identify with Hemingway's Old Man of the Sea or Dickens' Scrooge. Women's epic challenges are most often "other"-oriented. The many remarkable things we do are not often to prove ourselves, but to improve the lot of others. The welfare of the family, the community, and increasingly the planet, are places where we prove our women's selves.

Our thirty-thousand-year-old civilization has been under the exclusive control of the Father God for a mere six thousand years. His minions have seen fit to deny a voice to women. During our silence the planet has been brought to the edge of destruction. It is time to reevaluate our life on Earth. New paradigms for human interaction are needed, and these must *not* include war as a way to solve problems or acquire status.

If humankind is to survive into the future we must renew our covenant with the Earth. It can be argued that the values which must be restored as guiding principles are feminine values. George Santayana cautioned that those who do not remember the past are condemned to repeat it. The well-being of Earth must again be entrusted to the care and nurture of partnership societies made up of caring women and men.

As an elderly female seeking wholeness, I must choose what kind of an elderly female I want to be, and *how* to be that elderly female human being on Planet Earth. How can I repay Earth for the lifelong blessings of food, shelter, light and beauty? What gifts can I return to Her? What does She need? How can I help?

When one thinks on behalf of Earth, there are no problems with immortality. Earth endures. She cradles, clothes and feeds us generation after generation. She generates the latest fashions. She is the only store in town. If Earth doesn't have it among her treasures it isn't available. Too many in our generation, for whatever reasons, have come too far, too long, too fast without remembering to think on Earth's behalf. The full flowering of Her mysteries is waiting for us to discover. Our challenge is to believe in our own power. As Elders, but most especially as women, we are here because we are needed in the great scheme of things.

This book contains observations and suggestions on how we as individuals can be healthy, wealthy and wise. It also talks about some of the innovations we can put together out of our experience that will enable us to assume our responsibility now, and claim the rightful place of older women in creating the harmony the human family requires. We have the power to link our present needs to an ancient way—to find a flow which is meaningful but has gone underground to survive. Older women may be the natural dowsers to recover the river. To begin the adventure, vow to be true to yourself. You will not then disadvantage others.

Whatever else we include in our personal assessment, we shall find our strength through knowing we are all in this together. We are united by *Time*—Time the jailer, Time the healer. When we are old we are without nationality, color, creed, social position, gender preference or fame; we are merely old, molded by the Time we have shared. Prejudice will fall away even from those most content with their accustomed privileges. In the years ahead we will accept the help of kindly hands and friendly faces, and the comfort they bring us, because we know these to be the most valuable gifts we can receive.

Growing old is a mystery which is always ahead. It reminds me of how, as a young girl, I tried furtively—almost desperately—to discover the forbidden knowledge of love and sex. Now that growing old is what I most need to know, I find it enfolded in similar taboos. Hidden or denied, the truth is clear. We will age—it lies ahead for every living thing in this era as in every other. Aging seems far preferable to the alternative. It is my experience that it is filled with unexpected treasures, with joy and discovery, and with love. May each personal journey be enriched with contentment and years of kindness. We are Amazing Grays!

CHAPTER 2

SOMEDAY I'LL FIND YOU

W e need a name for each other. There are about 23 million women in North America over age sixty-five. We share a space in time, have lived through similar experiences, have needs related to our age, and look ahead with both fear and anticipation. It would be easier to think of shared circumstances if we had a "bunch" name, some way to refer to groups of individuals who share common characteristics.

I don't intend to say *old* women. *Seniors* is handy but colorless, and includes both women and men. It carries meanings which imply an end point. To say *mature women* seems inadequate, for who is ever mature? *Lady* sounds very formal, and may be something of a misnomer for some of us. The nonprofessional use of *Madam* doesn't feel quite right unless spoken in French and *mesdames* seems strange. I cannot bring myself to say, "my *fellow women.*" We have to name ourselves.

My Grandmother was a lady
My mother was one of the girls

I am a woman
My daughter is a doctor.
　　　—heard at a writers' meeting in Tacoma

The English language is stacked against women, or more accurately, it is constructed *without* women. Most names for jobs and professions have some sort of "he" word with it. Chairman, salesman, fisherman, etc. I don't feel quite right with *sisters*. Sounds more appropriate for church or union hall. Besides, sisters have special names like Jean and Pinkie and Sally.

For an informal name I have decided to call us *Age Mates*. It is handy and easy to use. It is borrowed from an Ibo custom told to me years ago by a Biafran student when his nation was struggling, unsuccessfully, to be born. In his culture everyone belongs to a special group. At birth each child becomes part of an age group whose other members, male and female, are about the same age.

Ibo Age Mates play together, start school together, study, get married at about the same time of life, become parents and share the experience of raising their families. As time goes by they grow old together. In maturity they become counselors, elders respected for their experience and their memories. In the traditional culture old women are particularly honored. They serve the community as healers, arbitrators, peace makers and peace keepers. But that's ahead of the story.

Ibo Age Mates reinforce each other. We might call them support groups with the important difference that the groups need not be organized—they just are. They have shared life together, danced the same dances, chanted the same prayers, wept and laughed through their years. In old age they are accorded the group's respect. Many of us might well covet the continuity of their lives.

In North American culture we are often scattered, adrift from old friends and familiar places. I think just being here makes us Age Mates too. If you will accept the term, we senior women have a non-sexist, easy-to-use, all-purpose name with which to refer to one another. Sure beats "little old lady," hey, Age Mates?

Those Age Mates far away in Africa have an answer for another problem—loneliness. I know from personal experience and many conversations that loneliness is common to nearly all of us, at least part of the time. We often feel alone and out of touch with our roots or left alone in unfamiliar places.

The absence of community is keenly felt by many these days. Being old and alone is deeply feared. Isolation takes your power away. One of the first things any oppressor does is to separate people from one another. An individual who belongs to a group is less likely to be victimized. That is why, for example, many writers support a group called PEN, whose task is to advocate on behalf of imprisoned writers everywhere. Being together for reinforcement, for the sake of a larger issue, or working together toward a common goal are positive ways to create community.

Individually we will be more secure, less lonely and less isolated when we find a community of Age Mates. We are more self-sufficient when we cultivate acquaintances we can phone, consult and meet for a laugh, a movie, an adventure, or just being together. A network of friendly Age Mates would help us all to reach out and offer support to one another.

A friend recently phoned to ask what was needed to set up a group of Amazing Grays. Only two things, I told her: a venue and an extrovert. A bunch of Age Mates doesn't require an official organizer to get started. Haven't we all organized a PTA, a Farm Women's group, a Faculty Wives project, a pack of Cub Scouts? We know how to do this; all we need is an excuse. One person can phone friends or neighbors, invite them in to talk about a book or situation of interest, create an informal time to share laughter, play cards or just find out if everyone is all right. It is far from a new idea. Our grandmothers did this in their sewing circles and quilting bees. Sharing our lives is what Age Mates are about.

Some of the places to find each other are in the excellent

recreation centers which offer senior programs. Most communities have them, as do many churches. These provide a different sort of pleasure than more casual neighborhood contacts. We need both.

Interests change as we grow older. Studies report that older women generally prefer a few good friends, seen fairly regularly on an informal basis. These are friends in whom we can confide and to whom we can show off grandchildren's pictures. There is no need to be fashionable, compete for attention, pay tuition or perform a set task. Wherever friends are found is a good place to be.

Our generation is more or less conditioned to look to men for support or approval, but not all of us will have men as partners as we grow older. Thirty-two percent of us live alone. We outnumber men five to two. For me, life has become richer and more interesting as I come to treasure the friendship of women my own age—all sorts of women. Age Mate women.

Getting acquainted is difficult sometimes. I often see interesting women in a supermarket or a coffee shop, but don't have the courage to introduce myself. Most of us have felt sad over similar lost opportunities, disappointed because someone we'd like to meet vanished before we could figure out a way to talk to her. For the extroverts among us, I beg you, make the first move. Those of us who are shy will need to find another way.

Remember those clubs our children invented—with passwords and secret codes? Let's invent an adult version. It would be great to have some sort of salute, or a symbol, or a secret *Supermam* ring to signal our willingness to talk, to share a cup of tea and maybe, in time, to become fast friends.

There is a delightful poem by Jenny Joseph that nearly everyone has heard of—the one that says, "When I am an old woman I shall wear purple ..." Perhaps that is an idea we could use. A purple scarf, a ribbon tied on your handbag, maybe a purple hat or feather—or violets in the springtime. If we did something as simple as that, we would have an immediate topic of conversation. Maybe both of us have read *Old and Smart* and could chew over what the author says, if nothing else. Quite a few groups are doing this, and a dozen or so have invited me to share their meetings.

Until we discover a better way, look into the eyes of the Age Mates you encounter and smile. Look for that sacred spark which unites women, lets us know we share life and place and time together. We each have been touched by the moon. Ancient threads of kinship, woven with a secret knowledge of woman's mysteries, unite us. Few have had the privilege of exploring such ideas, but we can change that now that we are old and wear purple.

We *see* each other all the time—in stores, banks, buses, doctors' offices and so on, but we rarely speak. We could change our isolation into community. When each of us, in our own good time, is ready to extend a cautious greeting from the safety of our cocoons, things will begin to happen. Pleasant life-enhancing, helpful things.

If you don't feel right about inviting people to your home, there are other possibilities. Make arrangements to gather at a restaurant or bookstore. Get together to discuss a particular idea or magazine article, read poems and stories. Take up a cause you share. Decide together what interests you. You'll find places to meet in library, church or community center, space to accommodate six, eight or twelve women without charge. We can build networks of friends within our own neighborhoods, create the community that so many of us feel is absent from the sisterhood of women. This is a new age of opportunity, a time to try new ways of doing and being. This is the only time we have. We need Age Mates to share it with us. Pot luck, anyone?

CHAPTER 3

OUR LIFE

I got through today, but what will I do for the next twenty years?   —Age Mate, 59

Recognize that feeling? An attractive, talented woman in her late fifties gazed past the portraits of three young people in graduation gowns and a grandly framed picture of a smiling child. She said: "I can't think of anything to do. Nobody needs me any more." Another woman said, "I used to plot to get an hour for myself but what do you do with whole days?"

The feeling, which comes too often to older women, is accompanied by a vague, dull ache, mixed with disappointment, boredom and low energy. Magazine articles call it the "empty nest syndrome." Others dismiss us with, "You'll get over it" or "It's just your change of life." It may be all those things but few understand the real pain and anguish it disguises.

It is, I believe, the mature woman's version of what Betty Friedan described in her 1957 book, *The Feminine Mystique*. Remember the furor this book caused nearly forty years ago? She dared tamper with the iron girdle of social custom and talked about the years of postwar suppression endured by many women in

North America, most of whom were miserable in the prescribed—indeed, artificial—role of "happy homemaker." Friedan called it "the problem that has no name."

Women who questioned their female role in any way were not to be tolerated. Husbands would say emphatically, "My wife doesn't work!!" And the cage was so grand, so firmly built, so new and well-furnished that complaints seemed ungrateful or selfish. Our very lives were distorted to make wifely obedience conform to galloping consumerism. There were all those things we "wanted" and had to "have." Frustrated husbands were heard to ask, "What *more* do you want?" Wives didn't know. We felt very alone and didn't know why.

In the turmoil of those postwar years, emotional breakdowns were frequent among women in their twenties and thirties. One friend of mine simply took to her bed for weeks at a time. Alcoholism became more common. Two friends chose suicide as the escape, as did many other women in their forties and fifties. Housewives monopolized doctors' time and failed to provide strong role models for their sons and daughters. Millions of young mothers stopped their growth and education far short of their potential. It can be claimed that the development of feminism is directly related to the dissatisfaction with women's role as our daughters perceived it. "I don't want to be like Mom," was the cry. Too many of us were buried alive in those consumer-crazy postwar years. Some of us are not yet free of our velvet chains, and thus we may still fail to know ourselves. The events which shaped us are profound and powerful. It is easier to understand why we so often feel as we do when we look back through our life experiences and remember.

The vast majority of North American Age Mates born between 1900 and 1930 began life as small-town girls. Other women, in urban centers—garment workers, cleaning ladies, laundresses, some of them very young—sweated their lives away, underpaid and not unionized. Most women growing up half a century ago lived with mother, father, siblings and possibly grandparents. Less than a quarter of us live like that now. Our lives were disciplined lives, orderly, with hard work and well-defined roles for each member. A good many of us were raised by mothers with Victorian upbringing. We girls toed the line politely, especially respectful of Father who knew best, careful to use our "good" manners and always vigilant for our virginity.

As girls, few of us perceived a future more dramatic than that accorded our mothers. We enjoyed some temporary excursions into the wider world we saw in black and white movies. We envied and delighted in the adventures of Shirley Temple. (She is also retired!) We played house or sometimes nurse, teacher, secretary, or missionary saving the heathen. Mostly we played at being mother. We learned how to do domestic tasks, to be careful, thrifty and obedient. Directly or indirectly we prepared for that glorious time when our dolls would be real live babies.

Few careers were open to women at the beginning of our century. Both opportunity and encouragement to seek careers was rare. Every morning in school we sang about King and country in Canada, and reverently prayed the Pledge of Allegiance to the Flag of the United States of America. I took exception to some of it. What is "liberty and justice for all" when you have holes in your shoes and not enough breakfast in your stomach? But I would never have dreamed of questioning the premise.

During recess we skipped rope and played hopscotch, hide and seek, a dozen kinds of tag, and roly-poly with our cherished bouncing balls. Some kids, mostly boys, had bikes. We made most of our own fun. Our troubles and tears were often borne on the narrow shoulders of a teddy bear who never told anyone and was always kind. The category of teenager hadn't been invented yet. Mutant Ninja Turtles were blessedly absent and Barbie hadn't been born. A doll with real hair and sleepy eyes was greatly treasured. Mine was about ten inches tall and I called her Lou.

We organized singing games and played Drop the Handkerchief, May I? and Farmer in the Dell. We barely survived horrible moments when no one would choose us to be "the cheese." We learned about loyalty and formal organizations in Campfire Girls, Girl Scouts and Girl Guides, Rainbow Girls, Job's Daughters, Canadian Girls in Training, and 4-H girls' clubs. How we aspired to badges, offices and safe recognition within the group! Boys were boss everywhere except in those groups and Sunday School. We could memorize better.

We were careful not to let our skirts blow up on the swings. We wore dresses, bloomers, and long cotton lisle stockings attached to various undergarments by imperfect trusses, hooks and straps. Remember the mortification when someone began to chant, "I saw London, I saw France. I saw Betty's underpants"? Hanging by the knees from the teeter-totter bar was forbidden. Sometimes I envied the boys their wild, thrilling games of King of the Castle and Johnny on the Pony, where they jumped on one another's backs like bronco-busting cowboys.

The years following World War One brought waves of immigrants with new accents and new energies to North America. These were not always met with friendship or understanding but we knew they wanted better lives for their families. They worked harder than anyone. The parents struggled to maintain cultural memories and mores from the "Old Country." Most children struggled to be accepted in the dominant culture. I remember girls rushing to the school washroom to comb out their braids, roll down their stockings and push up their long sleeves.

The children of immigrants helped their parents become "American." Kids picked up new customs and new vernacular, and when asked, "What did you learn in school today?" they were supposed to answer in detail. For mothers in particular, children were a living bridge between the familiar and the strange. Children of very tender years acted as translators for the family, able to negotiate bureaucratic mazes by the time they were in school. I remember meeting a grade-three classmate paying taxes because her parents' accents were too heavy to be understood. I'd walked to town with my dad and heard the office people say something about "poor white trash" sending their kids to do their work. Tolerance has improved since those days, on the surface at least.

Childhood sickness and sometimes death were real to us. Remember dark rooms when we had measles because sunlight would make us blind, or whooping cough that lasted all summer, or diphtheria, tuberculosis and the terrifying polio? We took our spring tonics and other vile-tasting nostrums because we knew the seriousness of sickness. All my fourth-grade classmates got vaccinated for smallpox, one bare arm after another. The year before, Colgate had given us each a toothbrush and a tiny tube of paste—the first of either for many kids. We were faithful users for decades.

Most of the children in my town had chores and real jobs as soon as we could handle them. However we complained, we knew our efforts were needed, if not always appreciated. We did jobs away from home whenever possible, and earned what money we could. Spare the rod and spoil the child was part of the religion.

Before the end of childhood we began to know the facts of life: Depression, drought and unemployment. Any old automobile, piled with meager possessions, brought families escaping the Dust Bowl, searching for jobs and food. They came by the thousands to the hop fields and fruit orchards of Oregon and worked from dawn to dusk. We all did. By the time I was twelve I walked a mile or so, picked prunes from eight in the morning to dusk, and walked home with about $1.50 for the day.

Many thousands of desperate men climbed aboard freight trains, riding the rails in search of work. No women were seen riding with them. How wives and families survived these long separations is not well documented. It was difficult in small towns, but at least we could make a garden somewhere and maybe store some food for the winter. And there were wild berries and abandoned fruit trees if we knew where to look. I still cherish ripe blackberries.

Terrible as it was in rural areas, survival was next to impossible in the cities, as some of us remember. Jobs for women were scarce under the best of circumstances, always notoriously underpaid and constantly under threat. What did city folks find to live on? During the ten- and twelve-hour workdays, who cared for the children? There were some remnants of extended families in those days, but often the oldest girl ended her schooling and became the surrogate mother until she too entered the sweatshops.

Except for the very privileged, Depression children were conscious of the economic burden, and did what they could to ease it. Remember trying to eat as little as possible so younger brothers and sisters could have more? There were few if any safety nets and going on relief was humiliating. Debt was terrifying. Lien laws could take away everything a family owned. A new baby was often a tragedy. Some parents gave up or collapsed under the strain of providing shelter and food. Constant terror lurked in some children's minds, that they might be put into a bulging orphanage either from poverty or from parental displeasure. No one reported on the physical exploitation and sexual abuse festering in such places.

There was one family where the mother wore a wonderful sparkling ring, an engagement gift from earlier, more prosperous times. When family tension began to build, the children secretly looked at their mother's hand when they came home from school. If she still wore the ring all was well. If not, it had been pawned again to solve yet another crisis. The children never knew what the crisis was. That ring was as good an indicator of the financial climate as the mysterious stock market, which apparently had nothing to do with the kind of stock we knew about—cows and horses and pigs.

The daily papers told of suicides and showed long lines of men at soup kitchens waiting for something to eat. One rarely saw women or children getting food in this way. Even in those days women were said to hold up half the sky, but many of us know little about how they managed in desperate times. I watched neighborhood people weather the Depression in the relative temperate comfort of Oregon, but how was it in city winters?

Self-reliance was the order of the day. The mothers in my small town could do practically everything. They were role models we could understand. From backyard gardens women canned, preserved and stored against the winter. Relatives handed things down to be unstitched, turned and remade into garments for smaller people. Creative solutions were everywhere. My other dress in first grade began its life as dining room curtains. I loved it. The one I wore most days was skillfully fashioned from one of my mother's dresses, but it was scratchy. Nothing was wasted or thrown away.

In the bigger world, migrants were shuffled into collections of ramshackle huts called Hoovervilles. In Canada, Bennett Buggies—automobiles pulled by patient horses—groaned along the highways carrying cargoes of despair and hope packed in around children, grandparents and the family bedstead.

Eventually there were elections, impassioned contests between the "haves" and someone everybody hoped would represent the "have-nots." Political contests were active events in those days. American women were allowed to vote in the Smith–Hoover election of 1928. Canadian women (except for those in Quebec) had gained the vote twenty years earlier. My Canadian-born mother was instructed by my father how to vote. She refused to tell him whom she had voted for, and over the next several years she was accused of causing the Depression single-handed. That would have been a big undertaking, even for my mother!

Early in the Dirty Thirties, President Roosevelt was elected to help ordinary people, and incidentally silence the insistent cries for political and economic reform. It was an exciting time even for children. Roosevelt's New Deal accomplished the long-time dream of rural electrification. The Tennessee Valley Authority brought power to villages, hamlets and individual homes throughout the Midwest. None of us worried about the consequences of progress as we gathered beneath the single bulb hanging in the center of the living room.

In Oregon the mighty Columbia was dammed at Bonneville. I watched the water pile up behind the dam, obliterating forever the enchantment of Ceililo Falls, where for centuries the great salmon leaped high in the air to vault the falls and reach their spawning grounds. I'd watched the native Indians who came from miles around to catch winter food working there with their spears and ingenious long-handled nets. My grandparents got electricity on their farm soon after the Falls died. I remember wondering if anyone really knew what had been lost. Beauty and majesty were among the uncounted costs as technology became king.

Telephones with crank handles spread to farms and rural communities. One could learn everybody else's business by listening in on the party line. Phones and electricity began to shrink the world. About the same time lumber barons started cutting down the forests, skinning the lush hillsides so only a fringe of trees remained along the ridges. The trees were huge. It took five or six playmates to reach around the trunk of what became a wide stump. Four or five trucks would pass my house carrying portions of a single tree. Sometimes I sat on the curb weeping for the poor dead giants.

Inexorably the world was opening up. My dad had been a flyer in World War One, and one day he took me to Portland to see Charles Lindbergh. Lindbergh flew clear across the Atlantic Ocean alone, and here he was on the Pacific coast! I traced his flight on the school globe and marveled at such a journey. When his child was kidnapped I cried. The large black outline of the little boy's body spread-eagled in a forest glade returns vividly to mind. A huge boat sank and a dirigible caught fire, a king resigned and airplanes were shooting at people in Spain. We could see them screaming in newspaper pictures.

To kids with imagination it seemed like everything was in cruel turmoil. The assurance that comes with orderly lives in little towns began to change. Our fathers talked about war! Most of us said we couldn't wait to get out to seek excitement in the wide world. A few of us in our powerlessness were driven by the need to try to *do* something about the terrible events happening everywhere.

But there was singing and laughter too. We giggled hysterically at Little Audrey jokes and thought ourselves rather naughty whether we understood them or not. "Little Audrey just laughed and laughed because she knew there wasn't any safe way." Knock-knock jokes were everywhere: "Saul who?" "'S all right!" And so on.

The radio helped shape our communities. The family gathered in the evening to listen to the radio and we talked about programs at recess next day, especially "Amos and Andy." We probably knew more about Kingfish or George and Gracie than we knew about our own parents. Edgar Bergen and Charlie McCarthy, Bob Hope, Red Skelton, and thirty-nine-year-old Jack Benny with his black sidekick, Rochester. Radio shaped opinions about age, black people, stinginess, all with laughter. It was a fount of comedy, music and kids' soap operas. Henry Aldrich, Jack Armstrong the All American Boy, Gene Autry, Roy Rogers and Trigger, the Lone Ranger and Tonto, and scary serials like "Inner Sanctum" and "The Shadow." The heroes, of course, were all male. It was just entertainment, not role models. Except for my favorite radio program of all time—"One Man's Family." It was different. It dealt with real situations, and included intelligent females in the script. Normally, when girls or women spoke through the grill of the radio cabinet, either they sounded simple-minded or they sang. "One Man's Family" was a pattern for living kindly.

In addition to hymns and parlor organs, the music of our youth was glorious. From wind-up Victrolas with needles that needed sharpening after every tune, came the music of Jerome Kern, Irving Berlin, Cole Porter, Rogers and Hammerstein, and the deep, resonant voice of Paul Robeson. I remember the first waves of magic as the Big Bands came over the radio, especially "Make Believe Ballroom Time."

We danced in barns, in halls and high school gyms as long as the cardboard in our shoes held out. Whether we knew it was a real thing or not, everyone took the "'A' Train." Hormones surged to fantasies of "Moon Over Miami" and we fell in love "When the Deep Purple Falls." The entertainment industry helped us through the Depression and gave us unrealistic expectations for the rest of our lives.

My parents talked about moving pictures with real music, not just a piano played soft or loud according to what could be seen on the screen. Al Jolson sang "Mammy" in the first film with sound. Black and white was the order of the day. The first movie with a few minutes of color was shown in a neighboring town the year I was in the second grade. It was *so* beautiful! Wonders were bursting all around as the Depression ground on.

Movies became our window on the world. If we could manage to earn or save a dime for the Saturday matinee our dreams would fill with Hollywood idols. We were enchanted by the bright lights of cities and romantic adventures. Through the haze of the Dust Bowl, in sight of soup lines, we escaped into the lyrical love songs of Nelson Eddy and Jeannette MacDonald. We coveted the wonderful ball gowns of Ginger Rogers and yearned to dance with Fred Astaire. We committed our lives to a fantasy of endless pleasure in glamorous surroundings.

The boys went to see the serials and we all gasped or hid our eyes at the narrow escapes of their celluloid heroes. Girls went to see romance and beautiful clothes. Every matinee had cartoons. Mickey Mouse, that unlikely rodent, has been in the movies all our lives. We saw murky clips of war and killing in *The March of Time* or tragedy introduced by that weird rooster screaming out *Pathe News*, whatever that was. Walter Winchell chattered on like a machine gun of doom. Hourly newscasts would come with the next world war.

In small-town Oregon, school kids were perplexed but hardly troubled by the strange events in faraway Europe. Newsreels began showing millions of people shouting with their right arms up in the air and soldiers marched kicking their legs straight out. The boys used to imitate them. Bread lines made the newsreel too. The event that turned me into a preteen political activist was seeing men in New York pour great cans of milk down the sewer. I hated them. Sometimes I was hungry and in any event, waste was a sin!

Suddenly there *was* war—the *second* World War. The world wasn't safe for democracy despite what our fathers said. Men and boys signed up, sometimes just to get the boots. They went off to save the world from Hitler and to die. Almost overnight everyone had jobs. War and jobs came so quickly on the Depression that some of us were still making our underwear out of flour sacks.

Official involvement in the war came earlier in Europe and Canada than in the United States. While the bombers raged over England, in our unconscious minds we knew that America would have to give up her resistance to entangling alliances eventually and go win the war for the people "over there." Modesty has never been one of America's notable qualities.

While boys rushed to sign up for the National Guard or were drafted, girls stayed unquietly behind. But we could get jobs easily. At fourteen I graduated from picking fruit in the fields to working at the prune dryer—ten-hour days for twenty-five cents an hour! Enough for a *family* to live on! I started saving for college.

As demand grew and men disappeared, farm women filled in to keep up food production. After years of glutted markets and plowed-under crops, everyone everywhere needed food *now!* In addition to planting, tending and harvesting, women repaired tractors, drove trucks and buses and, for minimal pay, took on the workload of jobs they weren't supposed to be capable of doing.

Soon some women were hired in war plants to build weapons to win the Battle of Britain. The call went out for workers in steel mills, shipyards and airplane plants as North America converted to a wartime footing. Some factories were even hiring "negroes" where the American Federation of Labor would permit. Women workers were symbolized by Rosie the Riveter. Women worked fifty- to sixty-hour weeks in war plants. When a woman got her job she was often harassed by fellow workers: "Maybe we can't get over there to shoot them Huns but we can keep dumb broads under control." It was a very cultured time.

Pearl Harbor was attacked December 7, 1941. The US declared war on Japan the following day, and four days later America was at war with Germany and Italy as well.

"Red Sails in the Sunset" became Liberty Ships stealing silently out of port in total darkness, carrying friends, lovers and neighbors inexorably away to daring exploits and enormous dangers. Families were urged to lay in emergency food rations. Most did, and replenished them regularly into the late fifties—just in case. Even then some people built or thought about building bomb shelters. My little brothers and sisters dug foxholes in the backyard and happily played war for years.

In the evenings girls and women volunteered for civil defense duties or prepared bandages for the Red Cross, just as our mothers had done twenty years before. We knit socks, scarves, hats, sweaters and even baby clothes, in ugly khaki green. We planted Victory Gardens, bought War Stamps, mended our stockings if we had them. On weekends we entertained "the boys" at the USO with donuts and polite dancing while they waited, tentatively, apprehensively—in great need of tenderness—for orders to ship out. The times overflowed with bittersweet encounters. One of the top dance tunes of the day was "Don't Sit Under the Apple Tree With Anyone Else But Me."

After we kissed the boys goodbye—friends, fathers, brothers, cousins, lovers and husbands—we searched for something to do to relieve the terrible tension of waiting. With millions of men at arms all over the world, millions of women were "saving themselves" for absent lovers. We were also scared. I remember twenty-four girls huddled night after night in a college basement expecting the Japanese to bomb the blacked-out Oregon coast. Loneliness, anxiety and sorrow played insistent minor chords to the powerful, exultant refrain of total mobilization. The war effort boomed forward.

In 1942 I went to Maryland to get married, and found myself in the heart of the war industry. I discovered women on double shifts doing men's traditional jobs. They "manned" the home front, "womanned" dingy offices, and slept in lonely bedrooms. In war-swollen Baltimore, sometimes three girls would share a single bed and sleep in eight-hour shifts.

Our Depression skills were useful in wartime. We made do with rationing, wasted nothing, and saved—money, string, tinfoil, cans. We collected cooking fat for soap and explosives. We wore drab, skimpy, fabric-saving clothes. We painted our legs with make-believe stockings and sketched in the seams with eyebrow pencil. Someday we would have those miraculous, just-invented nylons. Our rationed shoes were half-soled or again stuffed with cardboard. We did a lot of mending, especially of stockings. Anyone remember those funny little hook gadgets for reweaving runs? We gave anything still wearable to Russian War Relief for the families and soldiers holding off more than two-thirds of the German army. We heard from time to time about the citizens of Leningrad, starving as they endured what would be three years of Nazi blockade. We heard about the Blitz of England, and a little of the heroism of ordinary people who sent their young children away for safety. Nothing actually happened to us in Fortress America.

After the Dieppe fiasco endured by Canadians, the United States would eventually relieve some of the relentless pressure on Britain and Russia by opening the Second Front in Normandy, France, on June 6, 1944. A neighbor got his leg blown off that day. He was eighteen.

The Air Force set up an aluminum recycling depot in a park in the middle of Baltimore. We were told to bring our cooking pots to be melted down for airplanes. I passed it every morning—with growing guilt. Finally, I took one of my three just-married saucepans and threw it reluctantly over the fence onto the growing pile. It was there until we moved to Utah three years later. Maybe it is still there. The meaning of SNAFU (Situation Normal All Fouled Up) was becoming apparent.

Men's battles are writ large on screen, on stage and in books. Men wear campaign ribbons, retell their war stories, remember their buddies. Except for the relatively few and often maligned women who served in the war, our efforts during those days were as nothing, submerged in anonymity, hardly remembered, rarely mentioned. The only things we wrote were carefully worded, censor-proof letters to distant soldiers. We never wrote history. I was glad to hear that none less than the memorable singer Vera Lynn has been writing an account of British women's part in the war. She would know.

We *did* work. The war changed our lives—briefly. Women got a heady whiff of independence in those years. We gained confidence and pride in our ability to do any and all jobs that needed doing. We met all sorts of challenges, filled seemingly impossible quotas. We cared passionately about our work, putting in hours of unpaid overtime. We endured dangerous working conditions without a thought for personal safety or protective gear. The morning and evening bus rides of an hour and more were where women met and talked until their bus stops came.

My Baltimore neighbor built Liberty Ships, riveting huge steel plates into position. She thought about problems the troops would face getting out of such cramped quarters. She made some suggestions about how to ease the situation and was immediately shifted out of the industry. As a last gesture, she scratched her initials and a message of hope for the men who would sail in the restricted compartment of "her" ship. When it was sunk, she wept. Every sailor was lost. They couldn't get out to the life rafts.

Women were not well tolerated by the men who remained on the home front. Since they couldn't be overseas becoming heroes, many of them did what they could to make life miserable for their female co-workers. One night one of the regular riders got on the bus with her left hand bandaged and in obvious pain. Over the next few days we heard her story. Her supervisor insisted she perform her welding job in a particular way, but she was left-handed and had to hold her tools differently to work on the seams. He decided to teach her a lesson, heated a wrench with his blow torch, and yelled, "Take this you dumb cow and use it the right way!" She reached for it. Her left hand was burned through the flesh right down to the tendons. The hero's remark was, "Too bad! Let that be a lesson to ya!"

Another girl friend—we *were* "girls" then—worked ten- or twelve-hour days, six-day weeks, sewing uniforms. Sometimes she worked on Sunday too. Her fingers were raw and needle-stuck. Quotas were unrealistically high. Other members of the 7:00 a.m. to 7:00 p.m. bus riders' community made guns, fitted shell casings, and dreamed of war's end and the end of double shifts. My job as junior typist in the Office of Price Administration was colorless by comparison. A mere fifty-six-hour week unless there was a deadline to meet. My duties grew to include everything from writing news releases, the Chairman's speeches and the legal department's news reports, to performing in a weekly radio serial that I wrote to explain rationing, price control and how everyone needed to do more with less. All on a junior typist's salary. I could also make five perfect carbon copies—with difficulty. Photocopying wouldn't be invented for another twenty years or so. After cooking our frugal rationed meal, I walked many blocks to the university, worked two to four hours at night as an unpaid typist and/or lab technician for my student husband, and walked home.

Sometimes there were rumors of shipments of rationed foods. After regular work, one stood in line, hoping to avoid another week without meat, cheese, eggs or coffee. Since I usually worked late, the shipment was often sold out so we ate laboratory chickens and experimental three-day incubated eggs. They were thought to be infertile. I continue to break eggs with caution. I spent Sundays at the laboratory after doing the laundry in the bathtub with what passed for soap in those days. I was tired for three straight years, but so was everyone else.

It may have been most difficult for those who stayed home with children. There was little communication with soldiers, sailors and marines in that war. Waiting and not knowing was devitalizing. My friend and her toddler observed a ceremony each night at bedtime. The child gave a goodnight kiss to his father's picture—a father who would never see him.

Germany surrendered May 7, 1945, and finally, Johnny came marching home again, for the most part greatly changed by either injury or experience. We welcomed him with love and open arms, letting the great fountain of emotion surge into life. Most of us had kept emotions carefully suppressed during the years apart. All of a sudden everything changed. The supportive "women's world" we had built on the busses and at the ration office fell apart. There was no one to talk to who might understand.

The change that shocked most was what had happened to sexuality. With our romantic Hollywood dreams as guidance, and after months and years of abstinence, the returning soldiers' expectations destroyed the only version of sex we knew. They had learned things in Europe that we would never know. We women had been expected to remain true, as in movies, and forget about sex. It had been different for the men. Facing death daily, they had other things to suppress. Few even dreamed that we would find the reunions difficult.

We changed too in another way. Despite war's excitement and glory, the heroics, gold star mothers or widow's pensions, every honest woman I know made a secret vow in her heart that war would not happen again. We hated the men's stories. Sometimes we threw up just from listening. War and memories of war are the ultimate male ego trip. Women who give life do not think killing, destruction, plunder, and guts spewed all over worthy of retelling. No matter which "side" wins, wherever we live on the planet, women are war's victims and our children are victims with us. We felt hope and joy when the United Nations was signed into being on June 26, 1945. Germany had surrendered on a spring day five weeks earlier.

I danced the end of European World War Two in the streets of Salt Lake City. The next morning's newspaper carried an item with the titillating headline, "Two Wheelbarrows Full of Women's Panties Collected from Night's Celebration." I never have figured that out exactly. Maybe I left too early.

We rejoiced at every successful homecoming, wept with the others, felt proud that our hard work had helped "bring the boys home." On August 6, 1945, America dropped the first atomic bomb on Hiroshima; three days later the second one was dropped on Nagasaki, and the world changed forever. Man could now destroy all life on Earth. Dangerous, destructive elements carefully hidden deep within Earth's crust were exhumed to leer like devils in our days and haunt our dreams at night. How much changed we do not fully understand even now. Japan surrendered August 15. The war was over. For a while.

We continued with our jobs and watched our menfolk relax into the peace of home. Then came the guilt trips. "Women Go Home" slogans appeared on walls and sidewalks. Posters pleaded tearfully for us to give up our jobs for "one of our boys." Eventually we were kicked out. Any consequences unemployment might cause in *our* lives was not considered. I still had a husband in graduate school and needed the job. The "boy" who took my $125 a month job in Baltimore was nearly as old as my father, a member of the most exclusive club in town, and spent much of his very large salary on races at Pimlico. He later became a senator.

We working women knew we had done a good job. Absenteeism had been minimal and complaints rare despite long hours, machinery that was overworked and often unsafe, and dangerous harassment. We had kept working despite the ongoing refusal of unions to admit us to the protection of membership; despite sickness, cramps, worry, fatigue. No matter what the problems or sorrows, we filled our quotas and were proud.

We were full of spirit, confident of our ability to do what was needed and do it well. We had cared enough about freedom, democracy, our menfolk and the people of occupied Europe to keep on working when we were ready to drop. Women of my generation were so important to the war effort that the moment it ended our reward was to be sent home and told to have lots of babies. We even did that.

Among the Age Mates I've talked to about the war, most are unable to recollect what they did during those tense, hectic times. Memories lie deeply buried in the debris of self-esteem, suppressed and unacknowledged. In spite of our years of devoted work, it hurt to discover we were unimportant after all. When memories do flood back, they sometimes bring tears.

Within the year of war's end, nearly everyone was married and giving birth to millions of lovely, shining children. For the next five years the North American birth rate was higher than that of any other Western nation and higher than that of India, Japan or Burma. The US was the only industrially "advanced" nation and one of few in the world where more girls married at ages fifteen to nineteen than at any other age.

From war plant to nursery, our work became the nurturing of our children, and homemaking. Industry took off without us, and created the postwar boom pacifying women with the voluminous "New Look." Remember? Skirts nearly to the floor, real wool, and colors? This was a welcome replacement for skimpy clothes and wartime coveralls. We went shopping immediately, whether we could afford it or not, and have never looked back. We became the guinea pigs for one of society's grandest scams. Housewives were to be the vehicles of economic recovery, brood stock of a nation.

A torrent of consumer goods rushed from newly converted war

plants. We rejoiced to have nylon stockings, washing machines, refrigerators, toasters, mixers, vacuum cleaners and kitchen ranges. There were hundreds of gadgets, things, gimmicks. All the meat, sugar, shoes and soap we could use. Everything could be bought. Even mangles. Do you remember mangles? They were a status symbol, the ultimate in useless, make-work contrivances that occupied half a room. Just so we could iron our sheets and dish towels!

And so began the emptiness. As prosperity grew women became increasingly isolated from each other. Individual homes developed into fortresses of self-sufficiency—display rooms of a husband's success. Babies, endless radio soap operas and the occasional kaffee klatsch, source of much masculine contempt, filled in empty days. Nights were filled with diapers, pablum, child care, marital fidelity and games of canasta. Many of us were profoundly unhappy and felt guilty about it. After all, we owed it to Hubby for what he did during the war, risking his life and all. We stayed home, secure in our lonely prosperity. Sometimes we wondered if this was all.

We read women's magazines. Togetherness was the big theme. During the war these magazines were edited by females. They printed stories about competent women with meaningful careers, seeking new horizons, giving heroic service. Male editors took over immediately after the war and the tenor changed completely. Now we became mere women—weak, dependent, passive, slaves to fashion, suckers for the latest household gimmick. You can read this in the magazines of the time. Women could only know fulfillment as wives and mothers, proudly displaying a husband's success. Any other goal was clearly unfeminine and undesirable.

The new male editor of a major women's magazine rejected an attempt to introduce a few ideas from outside the home with these words: "We decided against it. Women are so completely divorced from the world of ideas in their lives now, they couldn't take it."

It didn't take long to discover our assigned lot was dull, repetitive and very, very disappointing. We dared not say it out loud or even admit it to each other. Society obliged us to *like* our domestic lives; anything else was a betrayal of our husbands' hard work. The most profound insult of all was that you were not being a "real" woman. In a peak of frustration I remember fastening my eldest son's diaper with my Phi Beta Kappa key, hoping to remind his father that I had once had a brain. Didn't work, and I never saw that key again. So much for straight A's!

But women *were* good for something—as long as it had to do with home, sex and children. Women consumed! An example, copied from a 1950s advertising directive aimed at editors of women's magazines, went something like this:

> One of the ways the housewife raises her own prestige as a cleaner of her home is through the use of specialized products for specialized tasks. . . . When she uses one product for washing clothes, a second for dishes, a third for walls, a fourth for floors, a fifth for venetian blinds, etc., rather than an all-purpose cleaner, she feels less like an unskilled laborer, more like an engineer, an expert.

Some women had difficulty filling their assigned roles, always home, always available for sexual and domestic duties, all the while keeping their minds in storage and remaining somewhat glamorous. I used to keep house in high heels, my nylon seams straight and securely gartered to my Magic Lady girdle! We worried about our slips showing and dialed in more soap operas, tried new recipes, read women's magazines. And though we loved our children thoroughly, tens of thousands of us went into therapy, distraught, suicidal, unhappy, wondering why our lives were so empty, and blaming ourselves. In *The Feminine Mystique*, Betty Friedan quotes a woman in Ohio: "The times when I felt that the only answer was to consult a psychiatrist, times of anger, bitterness and general frustration are too numerous to even mention. I had no idea that hundreds of other women were feeling the same way. I felt so completely alone."

I received a note from a writer friend who said, "I thought you'd like to see the poem I wrote about being young in the fifties." She sums up the frustrations of so many of us and touches remembered heartaches. You may remember too.

Dishing it Up to Mrs. Corbeau

I've been watching
National Film Board films
from the fifties—
those persuaders of
air stewardesses and key-punch operators
from dead end jobs
into a heaven of gadget kitchen
haven for husband
bed for getting children
a sometime island
of unrequited fantasy
marriage and security
of two-way stretch girdles
with resilient garters
spanning social gaps
wear false eyelashes and breasts
because you owe it to yourself
to look your best
assure democracy

In the fifties I remember
mourning lost creativity
at the mothers-of-preschoolers meeting

rudely complaining of strangulation
by children, husband, daily triviality
food

Mrs. Corbeau from the Family Life
protecting the others from my impiety
drew me into a corner pleaded:
"But there's real creativity
in cooking for your family—
trying out new recipes!"
I've found one, Mrs. Corbeau.
   —Patience Wheatley, Age Mate

The GI Bill in the US put higher education and technical training within reach of millions of returning veterans. This one act moved the United States from a largely unskilled labor economy to one swarming with professions, skilled trades and specialization. WACs, WAFTs, WRENs and WAVEs had similar opportunities if they did not yield to the pressure to become housewives. But for most women there was no easy way to obtain specialized education. That continues to limit women's ability to advance to the more skilled professions and the higher wages they command. Few women our age have been able to build much equity in private pension plans. Many of us are now solely dependent on government pensions.

There could be an exemption from mindlessness as long as we worked on behalf of our husbands. Some of us did hold jobs, mostly low paying and temporary. As young women we used to joke about getting our PhTs. It stood for "Putting Hubby Through." It meant we would supplement the family income until he completed whatever life-work he had decided to train for— law, medicine, dentistry, welding, carpentry, whatever. Then we had to exchange the job for the trappings of domesticity. So we did our simple jobs. Got our PhTs.

Participation in the workaday world was acceptable as long as you didn't intend to make a career for yourself. As soon as a man qualified, wives were expected to cover their typewriters, lay down their drafting tools, shorthand pads, order forms or bedpans and immediately don frilly white aprons. We would look no more toward the horizon. Just as it hadn't been wise to be smart in high school, we were now expected to confine our intellect to the "kitchen, kids and kip." "Kirche" (church) had more or less gone out of style, and besides it was Hitler's phrase. But it meant the same thing. Out of love, and responsibility, I would cook some thirty-seven thousand, three hundred and twenty-five meals during my thirty-five years of marriage and half that many again in my present life! If I'd only hung out a "restaurant" sign I would be eligible for a much larger pension.

Thinking ourselves to be powerless, most of us did what was expected. Partly it was because we were tired and demoralized. But mostly it was because we loved our children and husbands and society demanded compliance. Many of us resented our very lives. Both husbands and society have had far less satisfying lives than they might have had were women free to contribute their special skills in those critical postwar years. Certainly those imprisoned decades imprinted many women with poor self-esteem and failed to prepare us for a good long life.

It was not coincidental that widespread political suppression was taking place at the same time. With half the population out of the way, their minds secured in petticoat detention, it was easy to discourage questioning or even discussion of controversial issues. Free women ask questions, and one of the first would have been, "How did our Russian allies in the war against Hitler get to be our dastardly enemies?" And "Why are we building more and more atomic bombs?" More importantly, women were prepared to build for peace with the same enthusiasm we had built for war. Wasn't that the purpose of it all?

By then the craziness of the Cold War and the fanatical fifties was upon the Land of the Free. A smart woman was probably a communist. All intellectuals were, you know. We didn't talk about politics or civil rights or say much out loud. Women didn't dare suggest that *anything* should change. Our opinions were ignored anyway, and eventually we were tarred with our husbands' brush. With Senator McCarthy on our trail, our family moved to Canada the year my daughter was born.

Canada was an extraordinary change from the hatred and suspicion, the prejudice and world ignorance of the United States. Hope returned as I left fanatic patriotism behind and came to wonderful, open, generous Canada. My gratitude endures to this day.

America, drunk on economic supremacy, entered its long night of decerebration in the 1950s. It was downright unpatriotic to think. Women were discounted, intellectuals silenced, blacks and minorities written out of the picture. Neighbor spied on neighbor. Telephones were tapped. The rapidly developing communication technology was turned over to ad makers, propagandists, and the CIA. For years everyone was scared to death being told we were about to be invaded by godless communism: "Buy your new car *now!* The Reds are going to take over the plant!"

Had women been permitted to enter the political process in those days, I doubt if "they" could have pulled the wool over our eyes long enough to invent the Cold War and imperil the planet. We accepted our political impotence and the world continues to totter on the edge of war. Believing their own lies and propaganda, men of power managed to sneak our countries into the Korean War, the Vietnam war, the Gulf War and dozens of little wars to prove their greatness and feed their greed. We let dictatorships stand, oppression continue, starvation grow while "ignorant armies clash by night" in a world bristling with profitable armaments. As citizens, we know better than this!

Suppression of the human spirit, male or female, black or white, young or old, is a costly indulgence. But somehow, in the midst of all this, the civil rights movement began to take root in the US. A black woman, tired after a long day's work, just didn't get up to go to the back of the bus. Sit-ins, bombings, beatings, murders, and finally desegregation followed. The right for all citizens to vote helped America take reluctant steps toward "liberty and justice for all." Jackie Robinson even got a chance to play baseball. With the Brooklyn Dodgers!

My first opportunity to use political intelligence came in 1961 when I joined Voice of Women. At the time it was the only group of any gender in North America that dared to speak out in opposition to the spread of atomic weapons and the continuing threat of nuclear war. As Three-Mile Island and Chernobyl would prove decades later, we knew in our bones that fallout from weapons testing would hurt our children. It didn't occur to us that we might also be in danger, or possibly subject to an epidemic of breast cancer. Voice of Women organized right across the country and were politely heard in Parliament. Only in Canada, you say? Pity!!

Even here the struggles were not over. Canada was just nicer about it. Women remained at the bottom of the heap. The banks would not give us mortgages or loans to start up businesses. Neither industry nor government gave us equal pay for equal work. Even when we did have something useful to contribute, it was not done in our own names. There is a clipping in my collection of stuff that shows me, elegantly coiffed, at a lectern. The caption reads: "Mrs. Blank Blank, wife of Professor Blank Blank, MD, PhD, Chairman and Head of the Department of Blank in the Faculty of Medicine, University of Blank, spoke yesterday."

We struggled with various degrees of success against barricades of uselessness. On the theory that one might as well be numb as well as miserable, too many of us went for the bottle. Or we were sent into analysis searching for explanations for our misery, blaming ourselves, deforming our children, and greatly complicating the lives of insensitive husbands. Lots of us became chronically sick with vague, undiagnosed illnesses. The pharmaceutical industry boomed. Women were pacified with prescriptions for large quantities of sedatives and antidepressants. Our very woman-ness was said to be the cause of our problems, and we were operated on a lot. I remember having six or eight D&Cs. They were worth the risk. Each allowed a few hours of oblivion and a hospital overnight away. We may still hide unhappiness in illness. It can provide a legitimate reason for the depression, boredom and loneliness that continue to afflict our lives. It is a heavy price to pay.

Just when we thought we'd seen everything, along came the sixties. The kids, now half-grown, said, "Don't trust anyone over thirty!" That meant us. Our beloved, shining children rolled up their sleeping bags, packed toothbrushes, called over their shoulders, "See you, Mom," and left for exotic places, or at the very least Woodstock. Sex, drugs and rock'n'roll! The Pied Piper of music led them on and away. Their revolt against convention eventually ended the war in Vietnam and many came home again.

But where were *we*? Struggling with unbecoming mini-skirts, bouffant hairdos, birth control pills and wondering why our husbands worked so late until they announced they were leaving—with "her" because they felt unfulfilled. Not all husbands, obviously, but a lot of them. Some of us had affairs too, with few permanent improvements. Who wanted to develop anything meaningful with a woman in her forties with kids? We stayed trapped.

Few of us entertained the thought that we *could* live without a man. Except for grieving widows and "old maids" there were few single-woman patterns to follow. Most of us had never even heard the term *lesbian*. Being dutiful wives and mothers was all we knew. Once again we did what was expected of us until women's liberation came along. Our daughters went out the door claiming more freedom than we could imagine. They made it clear they didn't intend to lead empty lives like us. Women's lib did not include Mother!

Women's liberation and reliable birth control methods allowed the sexual revolution to begin. We gaped, incredulous, at glorious, indulgent, carefree sex, and occasionally, mind-altering substances. Books, movies, discos, billboards, girlie magazines, sex shops, rock concerts. The Beatles brought their new sounds, new body language and new mores.

Those exciting ideas didn't include us. We were too "square," too old to start over. We mostly continued to abide our "unused lives" as *Shirley Valentine* so eloquently laments.

However, some midlife women did pick up the pieces of their lives and begin to live their potential. Some earned university degrees, one credit at a time, trained for new jobs, satisfied their yearnings to *be* someone. It may have been from necessity but what they did was great. They read Bolles' witty, helpful book *What Color is Your Parachute?* and stepped out to join the world.

I don't quite remember where the seventies went. Finally, at the end of my rope, after thirty-five years of marriage, I left home and made myself a job so fascinating that I forgot about domestic oppression for ten years. I discovered challenging, intriguing ideas filtering in from all over the world. Long after the children were on their "trips," I learned about inner strength, meditation, yoga, and a bit about mind-altering substances (which I inhaled). Lower-case love was everywhere; god was within; mantras were heard in the land and spirits soared.

So here we are in the last decade of our millennium and we journey on. All that is behind has shaped us for this moment, for this time of living, this age of possibilities. Now that we are old and smart, the only moment we can do anything about is *this* moment and we, with our wisdom and experience can make it shine—for our children, our grandchildren, but most importantly, at long last, for ourselves. It will take some doing but we can do it together. *The point of power is the present!* See you there!

Life is like a butterfly.
There's certain stages you have to go through
before it becomes beautiful.
                    —Susan Livingston, age 16

I've talked with quite a few young women while working on this book, and without exception they have said: "I wish you would talk to my mother!" I reply that is what I'm trying to do, and they tell me: "Please hurry! She's so unhappy, so afraid of getting old! I don't know how to help her, and I love her so much."

Our Alphabet of Time

What have we done with all our years?

A Aided, aired and acted

B Baked, built, birthed, bandaged, bought

C Carried, canned, created, chosen, comforted, cooked, counted, crawled, called, claimed, canceled, and cried

D Done, drained, decorated, drawn, divided, demonstrated, dieted, devoted, designed and dished up 40,000 meals

E Eaten, earned, erected, emptied, erased, endured, embroidered, enlightened, entertained, explained and envied

F Found, fixed, feared, favored, flung, flown and flavored

G Given, gathered, gotten, grown

H Held, heard, helped, hovered, hearkened and hoped

I Imagined, irritated, integrated and intrigued

J Jested, joked, joined, judged and juggled

K Kept, kidded, kicked, killed, keened and known

L Loved, laughed, lingered, longed, learned and left

M Made, married, managed, messed up, merged, mended, mentioned, marketed, missed and meant to do my best

N Nurtured, nursed and needed

O Opened, owned and ordered

P Played, papered, printed, pushed, piled, planted, paid, plagued, pitied and prayed

Q Questioned, quarreled, quieted and quested

R Restored, restrained, ruffled, resolved, recycled and renewed

S Saved, seen, sewn, stirred, scalloped, savored, seasoned and been sometimes silly

T Trusted, twisted, thrown, talked, taken, teased, torn, tied, typed, treasured, tried, thrust, toted up and taught

U Used, urged, undone, uttered and undertook

V Valued, verified, vented and vended

W Watched, written, worried and woven, worked, weeded, wept and worshipped

X X-ed out the false and ugly hoping to eXcel in beauty and in wisdom

Y Yearned, yelled, yawned and set the Yule log blazing

Z Zeroed in on life at this zenith of our years

CHAPTER 4

PEOPLE WITH THE MOST BIRTHDAYS LIVE LONGEST

Grandma, did you play with dinosaurs when you were
little? —Janine, age 5

A lot of silliness surrounds women's birthdays. It is supposedly chic to be coy, or demurely admit to "a certain age" as the French say. The Germans have a gracious custom which promotes even the most virginal of us to Frau or Mrs. when that certain age is achieved. There is much to be said for the Oriental age tally in which one is born within a twelve-year cycle, and one tells age by the names of creatures. If you were born in the year of the dragon, you will be twelve, twenty-four, thirty-six, and so on whenever the year of the dragon comes around. Each of the twelve creatures has positive qualities of strength and character attributed to it. And you can give your age without the telltale numbers so often difficult to say out loud. I'm a dog!

No matter how we dissemble, our age is crucial to each of us from childhood to a great old age. Age is a guide in accommodating others, in taking stock of time past, and in contemplating time that remains. Age is part of our reality. It is simpler to be honest and live with the number of years we have earned, and it's a great excuse for a party.

Birthday celebrations honor the end of one cycle and the beginning of the new. Most of us have created scores of birthday celebrations, but rarely do we celebrate for ourselves. One of the misconceptions that accompanies age is that older people never have any fun. A rip-roaring birthday party might be just the tonic to create a spot of hilarity. A writer friend approaching fifty (which seems rather young to me) invited us to a Croning Party, because from now on people have to respect her maturity! Among the earliest meanings of *crone* was *crown*, reflecting ageful women's crowns of silver hair, the crowning achievement of long life. This delightful, moving event, filled with love and laughter, so impressed me that I resolved to create such a ceremony for as many Age Mates as we could fit into a large hall. This became the Amazing Grays, and it happened very much as I'd dreamed it. The first year one hundred and sixty-seven women, young and old, participated. It was a truly amazing weekend, spiritual, life-affirming and a great deal of fun. Great good will and warm friendships were created.

If you find it difficult to admit the number of your years, a Croning Party will transform your attitude. It was the best time some of us can remember, a super excuse to celebrate. Ask guests to bring poems about events in their lives, the times they have lived through, or jokes that everyone can laugh about. Make a "this-is-your-life" collage from magazine pictures, have a silly hat parade, or make crowns for yourselves. A version of Trivial Pursuit can liven up the activities. Dance to drumbeats. Sing songs remembered from childhood to bring on gales of laughter, and maybe tears. Since laughter and tears are known for their healing powers, it is worth trying for yourself, for a friend or for a whole community of Age Mates.

The Amazing Grays was conceived as a one-time event, but it has happened again. Other communities have planned similar events, and the idea will continue to spread far and wide as Age Mates realizes the strength and joy we generate among us.

Celebrating *age* is choosing wholeness. In North America we need to celebrate. Very few ceremonies to honor life's changes remain in our impersonal society. Graduation, sweet sixteen parties and coming-of-age celebrations for young Jewish people are about all that endures from the many rich ceremonies that once ushered adolescents into adult society.

Birthdays are times to celebrate Nature's generosity and create Rites of Passage honoring time, rather than trying to slink into the future hoping no one will notice. How many of us thought to celebrate menopause or even evaluate our feelings as our child-bearing bodies brought that part of life to its conclusion? Such an event is a milestone in a woman's life and deserves recognition.

Let's not deprive ourselves of our right to enjoy mature age. We have reached that time in life we once could only imagine. At our age we are free to make of life what we will, to reflect, grow in grace, and give wise counsel. Let us gather dressed in flowing robes crowned with flowers and ivy, and bring new sisters to the doorway of our age. Let us sing and laugh together in welcome, read poems of praise for wise women, and dance a circle dance to the beat of ancient drums. The third age of woman is achieved, we have graduated to be ourselves, a composite of all our experience along the way—first as maiden, second as life-giving mother, and third as wise crone. We are repositories of wisdom. We are again at the beginning.

A birthday is the apex of one's annual cycle, the balancing point of the year. That particular day, however long ago, was your moment to begin the adventure of living on the Earth. Each birthday is a time for taking stock. Important activities tend to conclude or find their center around the time of the birthday. There may be a down point six months on the opposite side of the calendar year, but from that moment "opposite" one's birthday, energy begins to build. When your special day arrives, expect a flowering. Create a celebration around your year's beginning with a Rite of Passage, and share it.

I haven't always thought about birthdays this way. For some years I didn't even know which of two dates my birthday actually was. Sounds incredible, doesn't it? My parents had one version, which was much anticipated in childhood, but for reasons still obscure, my husband commanded me to have my birthday six days earlier. It had something to do with an insurance policy taken out with the wrong date, and if I ever wanted to collect I'd have to get the date right. Changing the date on the policy was apparently too complicated. It was deemed easier to change me. This innovation placed my birthday between two zodiac signs, wouldn't you know. It also robbed me of part of my identity. There was always a cloud of sorrow around my birthday. I told myself it didn't matter, it was ridiculous to feel unhappy. But no matter what, a birthday hurt.

In the last fifteen years I've celebrated *my* birthday. My new partner and I give each other informal parties when we can manage, and invite lots of folks. He gave me my first bicycle when I was fifty-five, and a wonderful calorie-ridden ice cream cake to go with it! It was fun. Being sixty-five was even better. The poems were sensational! Seventy was a triumph, and a total surprise.

If you are really shy about numbers, forget them. Something in our young-is-the-only-way-to-be conditioning tempts some of us to suppress the number of our years, or maintain elaborate disguises. If it gives you any sort of pleasure, go for it, but don't waste much energy. There is no reason for anyone to be embarrassed about age. Each year is a victory! It is an accomplishment to be *old and smart*, for you have gathered all that time living on this good green planet.

The distinctions among the seasons of life are blurred in today's society. The importance of actual numbers fades when we realize how many young-old women and men are around. More and more of us are healthy and vigorous, integrated into the community, socially and politically active. A young-old person may be fifty, ninety or more depending on one's own assessment. With improving health in later years, the saying "you're only as old as you feel" has become true. Since no one seems to feel "old"—not for another ten years or so—just think what we have to celebrate!

There is a simple birthday ritual to fix us in the cosmos. It can be performed alone or with friends. Find a comfortable place where you can see the night sky. At midnight, relax and look up at the stars. Wherever we may be we see corresponding stars—in desert or tropics, through thick forests or barren plains, at the edge of the sea, or in the Arctic night.

Generations of women before us have gazed up in wonder at the same stars, marked their cycles by the same moon, and millions more will see them after we are gone.

Fix in your mind the pattern of the stars, note where the constellations are located. On all your birthdays the stars will be in the same positions marking your place in the great universe of light. Adopt a star and make it your own. Look for it whenever you see the night.

The immensity and grandeur of the night sky induces peace and serenity. It reveals our place in the great scheme of things. Among the rights to which women are entitled is to feel safe under the stars, to be accepted without judgment. Create your magical moment and consider any positive changes you wish to make this year and in the years to come. Look forward without regrets. Think ten years ahead and peacefully anticipate your life in the stars. Accept that your past has brought you here and made you what you are. For some, a moment of truth beneath the immortal sky will be the beginning of a mystical experience. At the very least it is a memorable ritual to mark a rite of passage which all humanity shares. The mystery of the heavens binds us together in the glory of the night.

Many happy returns on your day—Happy Birthday.

CHAPTER 5

THE WAY WE ARE

*Stepping out of the shower I visualized a contest between
Barbie and the Venus of Willendorf. Willendorf was
winning.*   —Age Mate, 68

ound in the village of Willendorf near Vienna, this "Venus"
speaks to us from the Paleolithic Era. She waited in her cave
sanctuary more than twenty thousand years, and is among the first
of thousands of fertility figures found all over prehistoric Europe.
She is a small, carved representation of the female body—buxom,
full-breasted, with broad hips, her hair carefully coiffed. She speaks
to us from ancient times when women and men venerated the
life-giving powers of the universe. Faceless, she is the antithesis
of the body/face we are conditioned to admire, the vision that
leaves us behind when we are aged.

Body image haunts women (and men too) most of our lives. We
are never entirely satisfied with the way we are. Our culture
breeds self-doubt. It isn't an accident that the bleachers are full of
opportunists ready to create and profit from our discontent. They
come offering new potions, magic elixirs and exotic concoctions
which, if we pay the price, will miraculously stop time, turn us back

into Marilyn Monroe with liver spots. Our common sense tells us these expectations border on foolishness; our yearning makes us vulnerable.

> In real life signs of old womanhood are not supposed to be seen. Women are socially and professionally handicapped by wrinkles and gray hair in a way that men are not. A multi-billion dollar "beauty" industry exploits women's well-founded fear of looking old. This industry spends megafortunes to advertise elaborately packaged, but mostly useless, products, by convincing women that their natural skins are unfit to be seen in public. Every female face must be resurfaced by a staggering variety of colored putties, powders, and pastes. Instead of aging normally through their full life cycle, women are constrained to create an illusion that their growth process stops in the first decade or two of adulthood.
>
> There is an enormous gulf between a society like this and earlier prepatriarchal societies where elder women were founts of wisdom, law, healing skills, and moral leadership. Their wrinkles would be badges of honor, not of shame.
>
> —Barbara G. Walker, *The Crone*

The women of power of whom Barbara Walker speaks can be seen in some of the world's cultures. Ancient faces, furrowed with time, but serene. They hold their power on behalf of "the people." Consulted on important questions, these honored elders are respected for wisdom born of memory and long life experience. The faces are strong and kindly. They make no apology for appearance, no false attempt at beauty. The Elder is valued for her age. She is the traditional Crone, a present-day manifestation of the ancient mother goddess who appears as the trinity of Maid, Mother *and* Crone.

Most North American women are treated very differently. Our

male-dominated culture does not allow women an opportunity to prepare their Crone personae, and thus grant us time to make the transition without trauma. When women ignore the value of their lives, and gear their existence to the wants of men, they neglect their own inner resources, and are caught short by the aging process. Women are denied the essential later-life functions naturally assumed in partnership societies—societies where men and women are equal partners. It is not only ageful women who are deprived by this neglect.

> Our civilization needs more of the gut wisdom women
> achieve simply by living as women; the birth givers;
> comforters; observers of human nature; and frequently
> the sole fountainhead of warmth, color, pleasure, and
> stimulation that gives meaning to the lives of men. Old
> men are supposed to have acquired enough wisdom to run
> corporations and governments. It may be that, contrary to
> popular prejudice, old women acquire even more; perhaps
> enough wisdom to establish better moral standards for
> the world.
> —Barbara G. Walker, *The Crone*

My son told me this story about a Hopi grandmother. It illustrates a power we may not know we possess. At a meeting of several hundred scientists, environmentalists and government officials, the discussion was heavy. Accusations flew. Tempers grew hot. The meeting to solve problems was on the verge of becoming the problem. Slowly, without introduction, the Hopi grandmother climbed the steps to the speakers' platform, folded her hands in front of her frail body, and stood quietly at the side of the stage. One by one the speakers noticed and fell silent. The audience did the same. She said nothing. Quiet descended on the gathering. Arguments and disagreements ceased. When all was still, standing alone, she bowed her head respectfully, moved slowly to the steps, and returned to her place in the audience. The wrangling congress stepped back from the edge of chaos and changed into one of the most productive sessions anyone remembered. The Hopi grandmother observed in silence.

The true elixir of life is not to want or expect to be some different person, but to be the best person we can be at this time of our lives. Stay open to the sun and the rain, be curious about people and places, seek intuitively for the possibilities, and reach toward them. Accept ourselves as we are—and with the assurance that each of us is truly worthy, enjoy the adventure, gain the serenity and the well-being to which long life entitles us and, above all, don't worry about what other people think.

A few years ago, a major television network brought a crew of four to interview me. They asked if other women shared my opinions on women and aging. Delighted with the exposure, I invited six energetic, self-actualized women to my home, women with real lives, unashamed of being Age Mates. We had a lively discussion, filled with laughter and their experiences of aging. Several times the producer shook her head in wonderment that we could find life at fifty, sixty and more so interesting, so dynamic. This person, in her late forties, told us she was terrified of getting old. When the program hit the airwaves, our segment was followed by an array of unhappy women undergoing mud packs, face lifts, tummy tucks, and various other physical traumas so they would look "young." The program was a travesty, an insult to the women who had willingly shared their attitudes and experiences, and their power to accept their lives and get on with living. It is perhaps unnecessary to report that I haven't been near that network again.

The first rule of an individual's good health is to accept who and what you are, and know that it is the right way to be, no matter what fashion or custom dictates. There is no all-inclusive standard, no point at which a doctor, blood count or thermometer will proclaim one "healthy." It comes from the inside out, coded into one's innermost being. It has much to do with what mystics call being "centered."

You don't have to be sick to be old! You are health. It is reflected in the way your mind and body function, your belief in yourself, your wish to live fully and happily. Maintain a positive, loving outlook on the world. And it is all right to be eccentric. We are generally healthier *and* happier than conformists. Eccentrics apparently access both the right and left brain more readily than average people and make far fewer visits to their doctors. Dr. Bernie Siegel (author of *Love Medicine & Miracles* and *Peace, Love and Healing*) and his colleagues observed that pessimists may have a more accurate view of the world, but optimists are healthier and live longer. I have been particularly impressed and inspired by older women who, despite various physical disabilities, let their spirits reach new dimensions to enrich us all.

Vitality, and how old we look, comes from the light inside us. It cannot be smeared on the surface or modified by surgery. *Yielding to the temptation to stay artificially "young" is buying in to our own oppression!* Plastic surgeons, drug companies and advertisers are lined up to take advantage of us, to shake our confidence, deny our ability to control our own lives. We are what we are. Trying to look or behave otherwise is dishonest. It is also painful, very expensive and temporary. We need to give ourselves permission to be what we are. It is imprudent to punish the body to reach some mythical measurement. Our bodies, respected and cared for, are what we need them to be at this stage of life.

The jury is still out on whether or not weight gain results from the changes that accompany menopause. Some medical types intimidate aging women, telling us we'll get fat if we don't take supplementary hormones; others in the same clinic may say we are more likely to get cancer if we do take hormones. Apparently no one really knows. Research studies done on hormone therapy (HRT) in women over sixty are inconclusive, if not contradictory. Whether because of indifference among scientists, general ignorance and fear of the female body, or inadequate research, *the physiology of the post-menopausal woman is virtually uncharted territory.*

There are few studies on *healthy* aging women. Doctors give us their best guesses based on the sick patients they see. I'm not able to enter the debate with authority, but, like you, I can listen to my body and use my best judgment. *Our Bodies, Ourselves* and *Ourselves, Growing Older,* compiled by the Boston Women's Health Collective, contain a survey of medical information. In addition, the editors draw on experiences of scores of women from every walk of life. They discuss women's health and aging by listening to women themselves.

Listen to your body, and be guided by its wisdom. Think carefully before you put yourself at the mercy of pharmaceutical companies for the rest of your life. Human bodies, like other living things, are designed to be *well.* Nature doesn't create junk, and rarely tolerates evolutionary mistakes for long. We are what we are supposed to be! Our responsibility is to maintain the conditions for healthy living. When you recognize the privilege of being alive and accept yourself for the valuable person you are, you will enjoy your wellness—and accept body changes in good heart.

You may have noticed that your children are suddenly taller than you and that the top shelf in the kitchen is harder to reach. This tells us Barbie isn't going to win the race. Time will win. Nature is wise. Some padding of the curves seems to be the lot of nearly all Age Mates. The spine actually shortens as the intervertebral discs gradually compress from the effect of half a century of gravity. Tissues once spread over greater height must go somewhere. It goes to waist. Right? Since compression is going to happen, be gracious to yourself. The older body is more compact; the center of gravity is lower and possibly equips us to better maintain balance and body heat. Interference with the natural shape of our bodies can be dangerous—even life-threatening, as women have learned at times of fashionable extremes. In Victorian days some women actually had ribs removed to achieve a tiny waist. More than a few flappers bound their breasts to shrink to boyish proportions. Nowadays some women endanger their health with liposuction, extreme diets and silicone implants to enlarge their breasts cosmetically. It's unlikely we will retrieve the exuberance of adolescence or the profile of a curvaceous sex symbol. If this makes you sad, ask yourself how much discomfort a wolf whistle is worth.

Most women lose body hair as they age, particularly those who are fair. Once-fluffy pubic hairs thin out to a semi-modest remnant. Underarm hair decreases. For a few, head hair thins, and "Thank God I don't have to shave my legs any more." Body secretions may also decrease—saliva, tears, vaginal fluids, even perspiration can be less copious than in younger years.

We bear honorable stretch marks on belly and breasts acquired while creating our children. For some of us these never completely disappear. Many of us are decorated with surgical scars that also thin out. There are invasions of our bodies made while hunting for appendixes or gall bladders, or performing caesarean sections, and sometimes these require additional surgery to eliminate adhesions.

Bodies change from improper diet, inactivity, or just from time rolling over us. To be sure, junk foods, fried and fatty foods, irregular snacks and too much sitting around, especially in front of the television, can add bulk and folds to flabby muscles. Women are brainwashed about slimness: seventy-nine percent are said to be on some kind of diet at any given time, although 85 percent of North American females are within their normal weight range. But guard against obesity. It is hard on our self-image and dangerous to our health. It is exhausting to carry around the extra weight, and it is difficult to find attractive oversize clothes.

My four-year-old granddaughter was visiting after a long absence. In due course the adult discussion got around to weight. Having added several pounds in the year since we last saw each other, I offered by way of excuse, "I guess I got fat, didn't I?" Quick as a wink, she replied, "Only sideways, Grandma!"

An enemy of self-respect and the most common reason for putting a person into a nursing home is incontinence. The ability to manage urine actually controls our social life far more than we realize, and on top of that we are embarrassed to talk about it. Finding a bathroom is a constant worry for many women, young and old. It may influence where we go for shopping or dining, or what we do for recreation.

> Bladder control can be difficult for young girls to learn, and for women to maintain, because while we are being taught to control our bladders and anal sphincters we are also being taught that "nice" girls do not feel or experiment with anything "down there," especially with the nearby sensations coming from our vaginas and clitorises.
> —*Ourselves, Growing Older*

Sitting for long periods of time causes lower abdominal muscles to weaken as well as the pelvic floor and the whole pelvic girdle. Inactivity, particularly sitting, can weaken our ability to control our sphincters and so result in an embarrassing loss of urine. Several adult versions of absorbent pads and diapers are now on the market. They congest landfills just like infant disposables, but may help solve the problem temporarily.

There are two simple exercises that may help solve the problem in the longer term. The first is to practice cinching up the muscles in the pelvic floor. Called the Kegel maneuver, it can be done wherever you think about it—walking, sitting, standing. Feels good too.

The second exercise concentrates on emptying the bladder

completely. Female children receive stringent punishments of shame and ridicule which may result in urine retention as a fact of older life. If you have this problem, it is useful to take an extra minute in the bathroom to contract and relax the lower abdominal muscles. Expel all the urine. Sometimes there is difficulty in starting the urine stream but that can often be helped by gently massaging the base of your spine.

Drink lots of fluids during the day but as little as possible in the evening to help assure a more comfortable night's sleep and less pressure in the bladder.

Even experts seem to know little about the basic physiology of the female genitourinary system. *Gray's Anatomy,* the classic medical text from which most doctors were taught, and the one I studied from, devoted several pages to the male urinary system but contained only one sketch of the female. As many as thirty different reflexes may be involved in the retention and voiding of urine; twelve have been shown to play direct, specific roles in incontinence. Be sure your practitioner considers all these factors in your evaluation for treatment. And practice the old "squeeze and release." It helps.

There has been a dramatic rise in the incidence of breast cancer in North America over the past twenty years. This raises an interesting point. During those same years, a great deal of non-medical attention has focused on breasts. Women have often been judged on their size and shape. Breasts have been given vulgar names, emphasized, manipulated, put on constant display from magazine racks to the front pages of cheap newspapers. One would never know that breasts had any function other than amusement for immature men. Often women felt shame if their breasts failed to measure up to some artificial ideal, and far too many have sought breast enhancement from surgical implants, with often disastrous consequences. Could it be that decades of self-consciousness over our breasts has finally been manifested in the increased incidence of cancer? Women who have unhappy love relationships are especially vulnerable to breast, cervical, and uterine diseases, including cancers.

It is not always easy to accept love for ourselves. Conditioned as we are to place love/service for others ahead of personal considerations, women of our generation often feel guilty or accuse themselves of selfishness whenever they consciously put themselves into the picture. This is the time to begin the inviting task of considering our own needs and interests and thus live more fully. We are entitled, as the saying goes.

Now is *our* time, the first day of the rest of our lives. We have earned the right to be ourselves, to love and be loved in return. Knowing that love wears many faces, build a support group of true friends. Love and care for one another. Get a pet to care for, plants to tend, a tree to adopt. It may take time and effort, but it is far more interesting than waiting in a doctor's office for yet another prescription that does nothing to cure an unhappy life.

Loneliness is the thief of life. It consumes energy and leaves us empty. Like depression and worry, loneliness has been shown to lower the ability of the body's immune system to resist disease. Concentrate on making friends. They are sure to be out there looking for you. Put on your purple, and seek until you find. Try creative visualization. Imagine yourself with two or three Age Mates. You may be spending an afternoon walking, listening to music, discussing a book, reading poetry, telling stories, playing cards, taking turns making each other laugh, sharing a potluck dinner, sewing or quilting as in days of old. Elaborate entertainments are unnecessary. Being there for one another is the true value.

Enjoying your own company is also important. Feeling yourself worthy and deserving is another recipe for good health. With assistance from the library and our own good sense, we pretty much know what to do for ourselves; we have done it often for others. One of the first measures to take is a long look in the mirror. Get acquainted with that reflection. Accept it and thank it for carrying on through all the joys and sorrows, the stress and strain and accomplishments made possible by your own special body, mind and spirit. After sixty-plus years of service, it is truly remarkable! No machine could ever last that long in continuous operation.

The Woman in the Mirror

I've spent a lifetime attending to my face
anointing it, adorning it, painting it,
loving it, hating it, wishing it were prettier
more ravishing or different
And now I am bewildered
I scarce believe what the mirror shows
emollients did not buy the time it tells
and I, on careful study, hardly know it
What I realize is the stranger there
looks much better when she smiles
And, if I look with love the
goddess in me will smile back.　　—Age Mate, 67

If we *feel* ugly, or unworthy, unloved, angry or bitter, rotten things can happen. It doesn't matter whether or not we believe ourselves to be justified in our feelings. It does matter how much we allow those feelings to control our lives. Two survivors of concentration camps were asked by a third person if they still hate the Nazis. One answered, "No, I don't even think about them any more." The other said, "I still hate them with all the hatred I can muster." "Then," said the third, "you are still a prisoner."

If we wish to experience a healthy, outgoing life, let's stop judging ourselves, our bodies, and others. Instead of punishing ourselves we could use our faculties to appreciate how well we function, and test our limits with gentle, respectful movement. And dance!

While it is essential that we accept who we are, we must know the difference between self-acceptance and self-centeredness. Dr. Hans Selye, who did the original studies linking stress to illness, called the concept of self-help "altruistic egoism." It is different from being self-centered. The challenge is to find that line between an arrogant, selfish "me first" and the self-deprecating personality who sacrifices herself to do the bidding of someone else even against her own better judgment. Self-centered people are more likely to die of heart attack than the less self-centered.

An exaggerated focus on the self tends to reinforce isolation and separateness. Looking out exclusively for Number One isn't "enlightened" self-interest. It's just lonely. And loneliness kills. So says Dr. James Lynch, a specialist in psychosomatic medicine who documented the connection between loneliness and heart disease in his book, *The Broken Heart*. What he discovered is that the most loneliness-prone people in American society—the divorced, widowed and elderly—are more likely to suffer from heart disease than others in the population. He goes so far as to declare that the number one cause of premature death today is loneliness.

What many Age Mates know is that helping others helps them care about themselves. Caring extends into prayer. A recent study found that patients who were the objects of prayers, even though they were unknown to those who prayed, returned to better health more quickly than a control group for whom no one prayed. This finding also suggests that prayers for peace and peacemakers may, in time, reap rewards. *Take time to pray to the god of your own understanding.*

I follow a routine at sunset which may be helpful to you. My five granddaughters are all far away and I miss them. When I see the flaming sky at sunset I send a wish—a prayer—for their well-being, imaging their good health and peace. They know I do this, and they think about me. Lately I have added a prayer for the planet, for her healing—and peace for her people. Who knows what a worldwide surge of prayer might do for the well-being of all?

Members of self-help groups create a community for one another, and share interests and talents as well as problems. The group can help reinforce good health habits such as exercise programs and healthier eating habits. They may wish to travel together, taking advantage of special programs for seniors, take up a joint hobby, form a study group or create a special women's place. Friends help each other by exchanging experiences, solving problems, offering solace. Friends bring laughter and anticipation. We are there for each other in joy and sorrow. Feeling strong within the self empowers us to reach out to others.

As we grow older we can expect certain changes—in our hearing, eyesight, weight distribution, flexibility and strength. Many of us will have to be more attentive to the well-being of our internal organs, our bones, our muscles, our teeth. Some of us will learn to live with disabilities that change our mobility dramatically. But these are conditions of *aging*, not necessarily *ailing*. We must not allow our society to define us as sick, just because we are ageful. That's one of the reasons this book is called *Old and Smart*.

Age is never a reason to give up! Until *we* are ready to "quit" we must vigilantly guard against those in society who would count us out. "They" *expect* us to be sick, decrepit, nonproductive, helpless, miserable. "They" also gain profit and power over us from the ailments *they* define. Everyone from the local pharmacy to the most powerful multinational drug house benefits from sick old age. Professions in their legions are ready to *serve the ailing*, with research facilities, pharmacists, detail men, doctors, hospitals, surgical supply houses, and so on and so on. *There are relatively few professionals to help us be well.* If the majority of the population is convinced that growing old means being sick, then eventually, we *will* all be sick, and those who benefit from medical intervention will surely take advantage of our supposed infirmity.

The shape we show the world is only the visible surface of our real selves. Face and body gain beauty from the soul, which is a reflection of the spirit. From there we nurture the emotional body which gives rise to the loving personality, to creativity, liveliness, our sense of humor, harmony, ability, interest, our sense of purpose, love of beauty, and all those myriad characteristics which identify women. This uniqueness is more than body and bone. Age, color, beauty, financial status, have little to do with the "you" in yourself.

Without your body you are nowhere. Respect it. "Use it or lose it," as the saying goes. Make frequent opportunities to move around. Walk, stretch or change your position often. Try to exercise at least five minutes every hour to activate muscles, lungs and heart. If you are watching television, get up from your sitting place during the commercials and "shake your sillies out" as Raffi's children's song says. The raucous rhythms of soft drink commercials show "a whole lot of shakin' goin' on." During the yell-and-hard-sell commercials, reach your arms as far up as possible. This has the effect of closing the eyes and covering up the ears. Airline travel ads suggest wide circling with outstretched arms, breakfast foods are good for stoop-and-bend exercises. Commercials for sanitary products prompt one to undulate expressively, hands on hips. Move whatever parts of your body you can. You can get a reasonable workout from doing crazy things on commercial time. Expel the air in your lungs whenever you stand up. Breathing is important. Five deep breaths when going to bed is almost certain to bring on yawning and hasten sleep, if you can stay awake to count them.

Stand tall, accept yourself. Walk head up with a confident stride, and enjoy your life. Take an interest in what you see around you. Observe the changes, note the colors, odors, the "vibes," if you will. Being aware makes life more interesting and gives us greater control over that which can be changed. This state of being is not for sale, not available on prescription or videotape. Nor can one give any of this to anyone else. It comes from inside. Strive to live in peace with your whole reality. Appreciate the miracle of being a woman, the whole functioning of your unique being. That's the way we are.

From Starhawk, a founding member of Reclaiming: A Center for Feminist Spirituality and Counseling in San Francisco, come these words to touch our lives and warm our hearts:

> We are all longing to go home to some place we have never been, a place half-remembered, and half-envisioned we can only catch glimpses of from time to time. Community. Somewhere, there are people to whom we can speak with passion without having the words catch in our throats. Somewhere a circle of hands will open to receive us, eyes will light up as we enter, voices will celebrate with us whenever we come into our own power. Community means strength that joins our strength to do the work that needs to be done. Arms to hold us when we falter. A circle of healing. A circle of friends. Some place where we are free.
>
> —Starhawk, *Dreaming the Dark*

Affirmations of Maturity

I accept myself as a mature person
I recognize my lines and wrinkles as badges of time
I wear the crown of the Crone proudly
I live lightly on the Earth
I glean from my experience positive, loving memories and
    recollections
I perceive myself to be sound of mind and body
I actively enjoy the pleasure of playfulness
I am responsible for my own happiness
I respect and care for my body
I am witness to messages from my body and respect its wisdom
I listen attentively to my Higher Self
I rejoice that growth is continuous throughout life
I greet each morning with gratitude expecting only joy and
    refreshment from the day
I enjoy my own company
I respect my dreams as messages from an inner source
I am modest in my needs, and everything I need is available to me
I move with grace and confidence
I laugh freely and lovingly
I am self-reliant and patient
I use my faculties to observe with love all that passes
I gladly share my counsel with those who request it, and keep
    silent when such council is not helpful
I seek the best qualities in others
I am considerate and supportive of the young
I am honored to pass freely on to others the skills I have acquired
    which they desire to know
I am careful with the possessions, feelings and sensibilities of
    others
I honor beauty, harmony and balance
I love Life and participate in its unfolding
I simplify my life taking only what I need of the planet's resources
I treat living things with respect knowing all are linked together,
    essential strands in the web of life
I affirm the uniqueness of my immortal spirit
I respect the sanctity of life and the necessity of death
I yield my body in the fullness of time to my mother, the Earth,
Knowing she will care for me as she has sustained me through all
    the years of my days.

CHAPTER 6

GETTING CLEAR

Despite all the things that seem to be wrong, I believe we are on the cusp of enormous social changes. Ever since the Berlin Wall was torn down by ordinary people seeking to change their world, societies everywhere are in flux. The roles of individuals and governments in political, economic and scientific paradigms are changing. While monoliths of power have tumbled, others struggle to realize that they too must metamorphose into new configurations. Even as Eastern Europe struggles to clear herself from decades of restraint, North America is searching for a way to maintain patriotic fervor when there is no clear enemy. Nations which filled our history with wars and conquest now call themselves the European Economic Community. Citizens are speaking out to claim their identities, yearning to belong. Who could have imagined that even South Africa's long night of misery is experiencing a new dawn? The great Nelson Mandela, free at last, now president of the New South Africa, calls for people of all backgrounds to forego revenge and retaliation, and instead build anew through conciliation and fellowship. I didn't think I would live to see that day. Back in the 1950s I often sat in a small group of people searching our imaginations to figure out what we could do to help change the terrible injustice. In the end it was the people of South

Africa itself, black and white, who made the changes. All they knew about us was that we were with them in spirit. Still, maybe those years of boycotting South African wine helped a little.

In parts of the world, efforts are underway to soothe religious extremes as traditional powers are dragged kicking and screaming into a new era. Churches, abandoned and racked with scandal, are rethinking themselves, hoping to appear credible to the masses.

Something new, and not completely understood, is struggling to be born. It is a time as traumatic as when the Middle Ages gave way to the Renaissance, which ushered in our present era. A great wave of experimentation with "new" ideologies is gathering. Even previously untouchable, self-regulating professions—medicine and the law—are gingerly considering reforms and new ways of being to offset mounting criticism from societies in transition. Those who may be tempted to sneer at the "New Age" are hard-pressed to defend the poor judgment and excesses of the present age.

The main ingredients in this simmering broth of social change are the aspirations of ordinary women and men. They seek the right to self-determination, race and gender parity, cultural expression and self-government away from the control of monolithic centralized states. Technology and instant communication speed the changes. Now that we can access information from all over the world, it will be far more difficult to keep people down. With any luck I too will be able to "surf the internet" and talk to women worldwide. *Old and Smart* is soon to be published in Japanese! It is important to consider values and ideas from other cultural models as they press against the conventional wisdom of our traditional power brokers. This is a most interesting time to be alive, and ageful women have valuable contributions to make.

What we are beginning to know is that societies built on the dominator model, with power-over everything, including the planet, have been bringing us closer and closer to destruction. The great unknown is whether or not we human creatures can change our greedy ways fast enough. One environmental crisis after another tells us Earth will survive, but we may not. Our destiny does not depend only on what we do for ourselves, but on what we do on behalf of the entire living ecosystem—serving Gaia, the ancient Earth Mother, not solely our selfish human interests. We have always known this in our heart of hearts.

The most likely catalyst for these changes is the worldwide women's movement with its commitment to equality between the sexes. Half of the world's intelligence is held in the minds of women. We need all the good ideas available. Women, given an equal opportunity, will supply many important observations and ideas as we seek to contribute to restore our threatened environment. There is a dawning awareness that our goal must be sustainability, not exploitation.

The dominator model of society oppresses all life on Earth. The emerging women's movement energizes change and inspires more and more people to seek their wholeness in harmony with the planet. As women make their aspirations known and seek their own power, we must avoid the present model of exploitation. This is not a call for gender wars. We must lend our support to building a partnership society where women and men contribute their strengths and wisdom in equal measure. Ultimately we are in search of inner strength and nonviolent ways to define our power.

Perhaps the most urgent problem facing our species and the planet is the unprecedented growth of population which makes impossible demands on the environment. Population pressure will not be relieved until poverty is relieved throughout the world, and women have control over their own bodies, which patriarchy in all its forms denies.

Like a honeycomb, small changes and new social phenomena are forming, building from the ground up. People are creating communities to meet newly defined expectations and brave old injustices.

These are grassroots groups without powerful hierarchies. They gather informally to provide mutual support, to search for clues to greater understanding, and for the joy of it.

A number of women have asked me how to form a group of kindred spirits, saying that when they have tried, it usually ends up as a kind of gossip session, something a lot of us reject as a waste of time and energy. I believe this sort of disintegration can be avoided if we create a "sacred space" together, a place where we can feel safe as we exchange ideas, hopes and dreams, joys and sorrows.

Most of the women I spoke with, and many men, yearn to find spiritual roots more relevant to their lives than the institutional religions they grew up with. Sometimes books, essays or poems can be used to open discussion. When we feel safe we are more willing to explore what is known of other eras and other cultures. Women and some men are drawn to the rich mythology of the Goddess Gaia, once revered as wise counselor, the provider and giver of life. Under a wide variety of names she was worshipped for centuries in every part of the world. Modern woman, her feminine strengths dismissed, is realizing that something vital is missing from her life. To address this deep need we have begun to design ceremonies and rituals to reconnect with the Earth.

Where I live on my beautiful island, we are surrounded by the elements. Earth, air, sun and water are a daily presence in island life. They determine my comings and going at least as much as that technological taskmaster, the ferry schedule.

For thousands of years, our ancestors lived in harmony with the Earth. Here in western Canada, evidence of aboriginal people is all around. Their symbols are carved into the island rock. Family totem poles celebrating their relationship to the great trees still stand in remote regions. With all the ancient energy and history around, it is quite natural to be more aware of Mother Earth. We seek to join in this veneration as it evolved in the centuries before colonizing cultures denuded the hills and carved the land into fields and highways.

When I leave my house on the ocean shore to walk uphill for the mail, I pass deep layers of shell middens, evidence of the abundant shellfish that once lived among the rocks and sand. The first question asked by people who see the middens is, "Have you found any arrowheads?" I suggest they stand still, listen and feel, and tell me where one would search for arrowheads here. It doesn't take long for friends to feel the peacefulness, and to know in their hearts that this is not the place to look for weapons. The only artifact I have found is a perfect, well-used pestle at the base of a culturally modified cedar. This was a woman's place. Sometimes I imagine them climbing up from the shore carrying large baskets of newly harvested clams and oysters dripping with sea water.

In the search to understand the mystery in our own lives, and of our island, groups of women gather once a month, usually at full moon. We seat ourselves (comfortably clothed) on cushions around a circle sometimes made of layers of fabric, decorated with symbols of the cardinal points. Once upon a time, on many continents, our cushions would have been animal skins. We begin each gathering by taking several deep breaths together, settling ourselves within the circle, being here now for each other.

We light four candles, one for each of the four directions. Objects which symbolize those directions are placed in the center. The edge is decorated with small stones, flowers or other beautiful, natural things. We create an adaptation of what we think of as a Medicine Wheel. The exact form is unimportant; the intent is what matters. The purpose is to create a sacred place where we are free to worship, pray, cry or laugh, and in which we can air our deepest thoughts without coercion or the need to be particularly learned. I am constantly amazed at how articulate the women become as they tell their own stories, and how deep is their understanding, how generous their spirit. It demonstrates for me just how much we need ceremonies, festivals, celebrations and each other. The rituals can take any form we like. They can borrow from many traditions or be created anew. No script is needed when the purpose is to seek connections among the hearts of the women so gathered.

We usually meet in homes or a hall, but sometimes a circle will meet out of doors, among trees, or in a meadow beneath the moon. There is nothing to buy except candles, and sometimes we make those ourselves. The stones, leaves or evergreen boughs are collected from the part of Earth where we are. We bring the gifts of Nature and Spirit to our gatherings, and declare them sacred. We share the magic with each other, and return the magic to the Earth. If you are tempted to dismiss such activities, ask yourself what *you* consider sacred and include it in your deliberations.

We have borrowed our circle ceremony from the rich heritage of the Northwest Coast, in honor of people who once celebrated a life in harmony with the generosity of this region. Over time they learned everything about the plants and animals that shared the space with them, respecting the spirit within all things.

The *South* represents the body—physical well-being, self-healing, protection, courage and love. We place gold, red or orange items in this quarter—things representative of fire. Sweetgrass, juniper, cedar and frankincense are added for their rich aroma, and gemstones of warm colors are placed among them.

The *West* is the direction of the spirit—dreams, emotions, self-knowledge. We place blue, black or silver items here. Water treasures are in this quarter—seaweeds and roots, and also dark feathers, pine boughs, sandalwood and lavender.

The *North* is the quarter of the heart—purple, gold and green treasures, things of the night. In the area of the heart lie wisdom, truth, rituals, teaching and learning, responsibility and Earth work. Salt, soil, oak trees, redwoods and magnolia are here.

The *East* encompasses the territory of the mind, and here white, yellow and gold items are displayed. We place amber, honey, sun-ripened fruits, smooth translucent stones, lemon balm, mint, sage and lavender for quieter spirits. Here is the quarter for ideas, philosophy, creativity, meditation and awareness.

As we sit around the Medicine Wheel, a feeling of being in tune with the deep and valuable arises in us. I am wrapped about in peace. It is a place where I can simply "be." I don't need to know the words to anything or the right time to stand or kneel, and I don't have to dress in any way other than comfortable. The only requirement is that you respect the totems you contemplate, and be willing to see value and uniqueness in natural things. It reminds me of some wise words credited to Flaubert in which he said the secret to writing is to contemplate the ordinary until it becomes extraordinary, and then to tell its story. Seated around a Medicine Wheel, the commonplace takes on a quality of magic.

Flowers and candles glow at the centre of our circle. Women who have been meeting together for some time beat softly on skin drums, bringing us together with their pulse. Drums played rhythmically, softly, engender harmony with the Earth and our own heartbeats. The full moon rides the sky. And we dance with small steps, slowly turning the circle clockwise as the Earth turns. The slow drums are for meditation and communion. Later they will beat with greater energy. We dance away tensions, worries and sorrows until rhythm works its magic and joy washes through us.

Our meetings are by invitation, our numbers limited mainly by the need to keep the gathering intimate enough to fit into home or hall. The circles are primarily a joining together of friends in groups of eight to thirty or so. The women in the circle I attend come from all sorts of backgrounds, from different faiths. Most of them are mothers in their thirties or forties, some younger, some older.

There are no formal rules. Mother Earth supplies our text. Although few people even know about us, new groups come together in response to a deep spiritual hunger women feel. You and your friends could meet too, and build a ritual made from poetry and friendship. It will develop organically from shared experience and greatly enrich your lives. When I look up to the full moon, I know that thousands of other women in other places see and feel the power of the same moon. We are united in our womanness.

The first time I came to a women's circle, I was both enchanted and dismayed. Everyone was much younger, and I knew only the woman who had invited me. As we sat together I noticed there was no hierarchy, no leader, no president. Just women who exchanged their personal experiences around the circle while holding the "speaking feather," a gift from one of the splendid bald eagles who live on this island. One woman burned wild sage and wafted fragrant smoke over us. Candles lighted the four directions of Earth, honoring the four elements. I began to feel in touch with something very special in a way that had not happened since Camp Fire Girl days long, long ago in my beloved Oregon forest. I felt happy.

It was magical, but I wasn't altogether sure why *I* was there— not until the very end. One of the women in the circle said: "Betty, we want to thank you for coming. You are the oldest, and thus wisest woman here. Will you give us a farewell blessing?"

I was stunned. It was the only time I could remember being singled out *because* of my age. Accepted and respected *because* I was old! The experience was totally new. Tears burst from my eyes as if a dam of pretense had broken, allowing me to be just what I am. I held my head up, tears streaming, and prayed a blessing on those young women who have so much ahead of them, so much that I have already known, so much joy, so much heartache, and love. It was an incredible moment. I have no idea where the words came from; I hadn't spoken a prayer for half a century.

That first night taught me so much. I suddenly sensed the timeless significance of the Crone. She is the old woman member of the life-giving trinity of women. Once the healer and dispenser of justice when her name, long, long ago, meant Crown. Now ridiculed in popular discourse, persecuted in theology, dismissed in man's world as no longer desirable or reproductively able, the Crone still lives. She is our special model because she is us.

As we consider the possibilities of age, it is important to explore the idea of *old*, how past events have determined women's place in humanity's affairs. We must seek clues for understanding what has come to pass, find remedies to cure the ills of a world unsure. We can start by unlocking the mysteries we hold within ourselves. The exploration will strengthen us, give us confidence in our own true worth, and bring us joy.

Credo for the Modern Crone

Her Question
Her Discovery
Her Vision
Her Way

The Question:
Why am I here, trivialized by my society, with a third of my life ahead of me?

The Discovery:
I am schooled by experience and common sense, with enough love to assist the care and healing of the world even as I undertook the care and healing of my children.

The Vision:
To restore the role of the Crone. Take back our power to heal, comfort and sustain our people, and enhance our Earth's recovery.

The Way:
To accept the Crone, whom we shall call Elder, until such time
as we have rematriated her rightful name, enabled her to fill her
time-honored place in humankind's harmonious relationships.

The Promise:
As Elder, I shall reserve judgment, and hold myself open to
whomever passes in peace. My wide experience holds practical
suggestions, economies and treatments helpful to others.
As Elder, I shall assume my rightful place by caring for myself,
walking tall, maintaining my flexibility and enhancing my
creativeness in preparation for my duties.
As Elder, I shall await each seeker who wishes my point of view
and give without stint, the best of my life-knowledge.
As Elder, I shall accept the honor of my traditional role to serve,
help and love those who come seeking.
And as Elder, I shall add my services to those of the many to
assist in restoring woman to her rightful place. Age has provided
me with special powers in the persona of the Crone,
representative of the Mother of All, Earth Mother and Nurturing
mother—she who brings forth life and protects it.

Thus will the circle be completed so Earth may be healed and all
beings enhanced.
Blessed Be.

CHAPTER 7

I'M JUST A HOUSEWIFE

I've never done anything with my life.
—Age Mates, 55–75

This remark, made so many times, seems to be the occupational disease of Age Mates. Well over three-fourths of us have done our life work as homemakers. We have invested our energy, our creativity and our lives in nurturing children and making a home in which our families could thrive. There is no work more important despite the disdain (of some women as well as some men) with which a homemaking career is regarded. The strength and cohesion of cultures derive from homemaking, and ultimately, so does the survival of civilization.

It is extremely important to understand what being "just a housewife" really means. We are entitled to an honest evaluation of why and how it is disparaged in our own minds and in the attitude of society in general. Much of the depression among women our age has to do with the feeling that everything worthwhile passed them by while they were diapering the baby or doing the laundry.

Homemaking is multisensory. It requires us to be intuitive, sensitive, caring, compassionate, respectful, reverent and wise, as

99

well as able to see, smell, taste, hear and feel. It requires us to observe widely and refocus instantly to make unscheduled adjustments, meet unplanned needs, respond despite an absence of rules, regulations or schedules. Consider the child who scrapes her knee climbing into the car while the family is hurrying to catch the ferry's next sailing. Try to put *that* on your computer or in a business plan. Such situations are commonplace to homemakers and can only be treated from the heart with empathy. They require an ability to evaluate, to feel and act instantly and responsibly, and with compassion.

The powerful male-dominated institutions in our culture—the legislatures, board rooms, churches, courts and schools—exist almost entirely from the five-sensory perspective. Sensitivity to emotional currents is considered extraneous baggage because it does not serve the accumulation of external power or the bottom line.

In a powerful book, *The Seat of the Soul*, Gary Zukav writes that our society has loss compassion; our businessmen, military officers and statesmen remain unmoved by the plight of others in their determined rush to power.

It can be argued that civilization as we know it would cease to exist in less than a generation if it were not for the ongoing work of the world's women. Dependable, undervalued, underpaid and unpaid women pass on the cultural forms that preserve the status quo. We even supply strong young men to fight wars. Women not only hold up half the sky, as the saying goes, we perpetuate the very civilization which evolves beneath that sky.

I can hardly believe I'm writing this. I spent much of my life chafing under the obligation to do womanly things which I often considered an unfair and unjust use of my talents. Who knows, maybe I *would* have written the great Canadian novel I started the summer my son needed help with math. Possibly I would have had a broadcasting career had I not been obliged to serve dinner exactly on time during all my years on television. Or maybe, just maybe, I could have made a useful contribution to sociological thought had it been possible to concentrate fully on the theory I was developing in university. I left it behind to follow my husband. All sorts of things might have been, but were/are not.

I don't accept the argument that "you could have done it if you really wanted to." That notion generally comes from the protected or privileged who could command the help of others, or who had escaped responsibilities. Our generation of women was conditioned to see to the needs of others before our own needs. Most of us were wives and mothers first, and fitted other things in whenever we could. Had we not performed our humble tasks, who would have prepared the meals, done the laundry, comforted the ill, typed the manuscripts or answered the questions of the lively, intelligent children who came our way? These were our responsibilities and we performed them well. Our remuneration was board and room, and the satisfaction gained from doing our tasks with integrity and love.

Maybe society would recognize the value of our work if there were ways to measure it. In this society which seems only to value winners, maybe we could earn gold medals for the best lunch bag or compete for Olympic mother as fastest house cleaner, most efficient dishwasher, highest duster. Contests for best baby feeder, speed cook, most dramatic story reader, and so on would be patently ridiculous, but shouldn't be more difficult to judge than hundredth-of-a-second victories on ski slope or race track.

The five-sensory society values scores and competition above integrity, excellence or truth. Because women's work depends on multisensory choices, one woman's work cannot reasonably be proclaimed as better than another's. A homemaker is required to do her best at all times, in a wide variety of endeavors and circumstances, not merely in preparation for moments of glory. We succeed at our tasks through love, and by creating co-operation and harmony, not by beating out the competition.

Matters of social substance, called "motherhood issues," are often dismissed by the dominator society. They have to do with the quality of life. Power is not readily acquired through them, and hence they are deemed to have little measurable value. But undervaluing women's work does not alter the truth—that culture and civilization exist because someone, in the overwhelming majority of cases, women—cared for its daily needs. Someone attended to "motherhood issues."

We share this work with women all over the world. Despite the trend to multinational control of agribusiness, the United Nations has estimated that nine out of every ten pounds of food consumed by the world's families have been produced by women! And creating the conditions for human well-being, the intermediary between production and use is generally a woman. Writing in the *New Internationalist*, Debbie Taylor says:

> The magazine's message was then (1974) as it is today:
> that "women hold up half the sky and a great deal more
> besides" and that development will at best hobble along
> until women's disproportionate contribution to the work,
> wealth and well-being of their communities is both
> recognized and rewarded.

The quality of a culture or a civilization depends largely on the competence of its women. It is better for everyone when every woman is healthy, literate, educated and free to make decisions. Then she is empowered to perform her duties to the benefit of all, including herself. She will give birth to healthier children, nurture them more ably, educate them to assume appropriate responsibilities, and the culture will thrive. Women impoverished in body, mind and spirit are less able to transmit the culture let alone move it into higher realms. The position of women within a country is roughly equivalent to a country's standing among the nations of the world.

Most women in North America differ from sisters overseas in

the vast amount of resources at our command, but not in purpose or intent. Unhappy or underprivileged mothers, here as everywhere, struggle to raise their children within their limitations. If ever there need be an argument for a guaranteed annual wage, it is in the eyes of women and children waiting in line at the food banks—anywhere in the world. We can only imagine the anguish of women in less affluent countries as they struggle to care for their children amid the misery of war and famine.

The United Nations attributed the rapid postwar recovery of Japan and Germany largely to the fact that the female population was educated. A nation thrives when women with their children are able to function to the best of their ability. We can only imagine how much more satisfying life will be when women have equal opportunities to incorporate their best qualities into the life of the society. We can surmise through scraps of history that a world where women are granted equality may be less bloody, less torn by warlike emotions of greed, hatred, ambition, cruelty, and power-over. We are peaceful not because we are afraid to fight. We fiercely defend our young. But we have *different* priorities, different feelings. We have children to care for, men to support, elderly to comfort, and gardens to grow. Women work from all their senses, including the heart.

Ozymandias

I met a traveller from an antique land
Who said: "Two vast and trunkless legs of stone
Stand in the desert. Near them, on the sand,
Half sunk, a shattered visage lies, whose frown,
And wrinkled lip, and sneer of cold command,
Tell that its sculptor well those passions read."
"My name is Ozymandias, king of kings:
Look on my works, ye Mighty, and despair!"
Nothing beside remains. Round the decay

Of that colossal wreck, boundless and bare
The lone and level sands stretch far away.
—Percy Bysshe Shelley, 1817

Ozymandias in all his mighty glory and cold command is dead, forgotten except for the voice of the poet. Culture, on the other hand, lives on, perpetuated by women who teach their children. Every other human activity—whether it results in social changes, business triumphs, conquest, inventions or settlement of new lands—will fall useless by the wayside and be buried in the sand without the work of women. We are strongest in peace.

Survival of our species will depend on how wisely and how soon women can effectively assert our influence on the world. Devastation and destruction as a way of life must change and will change as more and more men realize the insanity of their past value systems.

It has been said that we are less well cared for these days than we were in Neolithic times. Perhaps twenty centuries of war and plunder was the best men could do. The world has again and again witnessed mighty he-men racing in anger to the battlefield, eager to wield their swords, deploy their deadly ordinance, and bomb ancient civilizations back to the pre-industrial age. Women are never *that* emotional!

Men must take responsibility for suppressing, beating and depriving women. Violence toward women is cut from the same cloth as plundering the planet, building terrible weapons, and devoting extraordinary creative energy to ever more efficient ways to kill. Women must reject such "protection," and demand the kind of protection that cherishes and reinforces life.

If anyone thinks women cannot be trusted to run things, just consider whether or not we could have done much worse for all these centuries. Women, with their responsibility for families, direct their emotions toward survival, caring for the land we use, preserving homes and communities. I believe we are less likely to destroy life in relentless pursuit of wealth, conquest, greed and personal ego.

THE CULTURE-GIVER

Culture-giver is a gender-neutral term we can use instead of housewife, homemaker or "the wife." In my opinion, there are three imperatives for culture-givers:

- Culture-givers must gain entrance into the society and demand respect for children and the land.
- Women must be empowered to take on our responsibilities freely.
- Women must recognize our own values, abilities and worthiness. We ourselves must honor the spark within that gives us life, and employ the extraordinary talents we possess as peace-makers. We have a *right* to be heard. We have a *responsibility* to speak out against that behavior, anywhere in the world, which common sense tells us is *wrong!*

The woman who first suggested the celebration of Mother's Day said it like this:

Mother's Day Proclamation

Arise all women who have hearts, whether your baptism be
   that of water or of fears.
Say firmly: **we will not have great questions decided by
   irrelevant agencies.**
Our husbands shall not come to us, reeking with carnage,
   for caresses and applause.
Our sons shall not be taken from us to unlearn all that we

have been able to teach them of charity, mercy, and
patience.
We women of one country will be too tender of those of
another country to allow our sons to be trained to injure
theirs.
From the bosom of the devastated Earth a voice goes up
with our own.
It says: Disarm! Disarm!   —Julia Ward Howe, 1870

"Peoplemaking," as Virginia Satir calls it in her 1972 book by the same name, is a top-priority job. It demands the care and attention of both women and men. Happily, changes are underway. We are beginning to see bright, wholesome, healthy children raised by couples who achieve supportive balance between the sexes. True partnership families, with positive male and female role models for the children to emulate, can represent the culture-givers of the future. Permission for both parents to be the best they can be, as well as recognition of woman's true role, require new ways of thinking for the whole society. It will take time and much tact, but it promises great hope for the future.

As long as our culture is addicted to violence, a necessary part of our work as culture-givers is to be vigilant peacemakers. I cannot hold myself blameless in the world's mess. Most of the terrible decisions which have brought the planet to the edge of destruction were made while I was serving coffee or repainting the kitchen. We did not make our feelings known. We allowed the decision-makers to ignore common sense, to disenfranchise us as members of society. Men of our culture, without women of power to give them compassionate reminders, have gone on to unleash "the hounds of war" many times as they continued to plunder the planet. We must use our strength to help bring the forces of destruction back from that terrifying edge.

Let us call upon the wives, mothers, daughters and sisters of our senators, congressmen and parliamentarians, and join together. I propose that in our maturity, we no longer act only as the forgiving, nurturing mother, but also as the avenging Crone, calling the decision-makers to account. We have little to lose in such an adventure and our grandchildren have much to gain. Let us confront men who hide their own terror behind an obsession with "reality," who claim to speak with a scientific, objective, rational voice. Reality is in living, not dying for some abstract ideology or waiting for one more research study.

The economy will not suffer from conversion to peacetime. We did that after World War Two and created the most dynamic period of economic growth ever experienced. To begin with, there is a planet to heal, an environment to restore, and millions of workers are needed to do it. The sale and manufacture of armaments serve no purpose other than destruction. Ordinary workers, as well as decision-makers, have a responsibility to free us from this waste of talent and resources. All of us can insist on doing meaningful work. There is no room in this world for "techno-dorks" or arms merchants.

Freedom is the capacity to make intelligent choices.

> Do What You Can
> With What You Have
> Where You Are

North Americans tend to focus on the ends, all but ignoring the means by which we get there. This may serve industry but ignores people. Our competitive culture places esthetics, ideas, art, music, foods, and so on into small compartments, carefully separated one from another. It is done in the name of efficiency, but efficiency isn't all that is needed. Women know that life is a continuum, not a string of separate events. A carefully alphabetized spice shelf doesn't guarantee a good stew!

Too often we continue a practice, looking neither to the right nor the left, failing to see there is any effect beyond what our five senses can comprehend at that moment. That is apparently why the automobile industry continues to produce 20 percent more cars than they expect to sell, or why forestry companies continue to clearcut when there are better ways to obtain lumber or paper. That's how the environment got to be the way it is. When Nature doesn't show up on the bottom line, it doesn't merit the attention of short-sighted power brokers.

Even though they, like the rest of us, must breathe polluted air and drink contaminated water, people in powerful positions are handicapped when it comes to making changes. Huge self-perpetuating institutions are born, built and protected. Omnipotent ministries are established. Dealing with the budget becomes an end in itself. Red tape proliferates. Procedures become more important than the work.

These attitudes make no sense to multisensory personalities who recognize the interrelatedness of life on Earth. It is not sufficient to stand in the same place and holler for more money and more research while perpetuating old, damaging ways. There is no excuse to wait to do what *must* be done.

The first step is always to achieve wholeness, to do something with your life that satisfies you. Pious dogma will only drive the magic away. Considering that the goal is to *live* until we die, it is far more rewarding to fasten our imagination on the living part, rather than the dying. It is also more interesting, since there are no borders, no limits. The first small step is necessary before we can take the next step. Just as there are no two snowflakes alike, no two trees or sunsets or creatures, we Age Mates also are unique. There can be no fixed boundaries, since all change radiates out from a center, and the center is everywhere. Each of us is a center.

Women's many roles require flexibility, the ability to change focus from one minute to the next. Woman, wife, mother, cook, chauffeur, hostess, lover, secretary, bookkeeper, cleaning person, gardener, counselor, manager, and on and on. No wonder we sometimes lose sight of ourselves as *people*. But it is this very combination of skills that makes women's contribution so essential. It is critical to the well-being of the planet that women contribute their special skills to civilization now and in the future. Women are the unwritten half of history, and it is high time to start writing.

Workable ways to resolve conflicts are desperately needed at this time, and women excel at conflict resolution. A family faces hundreds of conflict situations every year, and we almost always find ways to settle without bloodshed. It takes a special talent to find a path between differences, weigh the competing interests and maintain a dynamic balance where everyone is satisfied with their piece of pie. That's what being just a housewife is all about.

If men could create a peaceful world surely they would have done so in the past five thousand years!

Over and above domestic peacekeeping there are specific actions we can take. Some of us hold stocks in destructive or polluting companies. The excuse they give for rotten policies invariably comes down to: "We have to answer to our shareholders." If, as shareholders, we make it clear that we do not support their practices, they will eventually change. We have nothing to lose. What can our dividends buy that is more valuable than clean water, fresh air, and peace for our grandchildren?

Age Mates like ourselves can take the bulls by the horns and insist on knowing *why* they are so bull-headed. What does it do for the power brokers to be so greedy, so ready to bend their talents to destruction and conflict? And we must talk to our own grown children. Ask them what they do, what are their motives, their values, their hopes for themselves and their children?

Let us encourage life-based pursuits, expecting the best of ourselves and others. Let the arts flourish, the pursuit of inner peace develop. Age Mates have the wisdom of Elders in an age when wisdom is clearly needed. We shall use our power to bring about those changes our common sense explicitly shows to be desirable. We need not question our competence.

So, as just a housewife—a culture-giver—our task is to use our common sense, to use our power as healers, the same power that healed our wounded children, and to become whole in a healing world, projecting the vision both outward and deeply inward.

It is time to cease mourning mistakes of the past and live in such a way that, with our help, Earth can heal herself. Neither we nor our grandchildren will be healthy in an unhealthy place. It is time to be wise. As the Talmud saying goes, If not now, when? If not me, who?

> Only wisdom,
> sun,
> and random cosmic stuff
> come new to help
> us on our way.

CHAPTER 8

THE HEALING MIND

A ll my years I've been fascinated by the paths taken by the world's peoples as we came to be the way we are—the myths, legends, arts, stories and discoveries with which we accommodated to our various lives. Every summer night at the lake I read my children bedtime tales about gods and goddesses from ancient times. We learned about sacred groves, rocks and streams, caves and mountains filled with spirits. We studied Arthurian legends, sagas from Scandinavia, customs of India, tales from the Celts and accounts of the myths of original peoples everywhere. Story time was captivating. It satisfied my curiosity and sent the kids not only to their dreams, but eventually on adventures in anthropology and archaeology and toward deep understanding of the planet which nourishes us through all time. During those long nights we were steeped in myths of the Earth and became aware of people's creative, even heroic efforts to understand the mysteries of their world. There are no strangers in the mythologies of humankind.

We came to know in our souls how firmly we are connected with the rhythms of Earth, the heavens, stars and the many gods and goddesses who informed the spiritual lives of the earliest people. We found stones shaped by imagination into goddess figures and placed them, as the ancients did, beneath big trees, beside streams and at the door of our primitive summer place. The children called the creatures they caught (and eventually released) names like Jumpiter, Minerva and "Crazy Old Tiberius" who, mysterious as he was, turned out to be an enormous tomato worm. They argued with me to keep a snake in the boat house because she was a sacred symbol to the people of Crete.

We watched pollen coat the world with gold dust, tree buds expand into a green canopy, baby birds fledge and fly away, waves scold our shore and heavy rains build small streams in the land. Eventually, when the maples began to turn scarlet, we packed up our stuff and headed back to Winnipeg and school and jobs where the gods and goddesses were scarcely recognizable amid the traffic and the competition of city life. But we had touched the infinite, and it remains with us—the ancient, honored oneness of people and Earth.

This sense had guided humanity in peace and reverence for an estimated 30,000 years until it was changed by the strokes of a thousand swords, the swords of conquest wielded on behalf of a single, remote, angry male god; the tree of life with its roots in the deepest earth and its branches reaching the constellations, gave way to the hewn cross. People grew accustomed to the subjugation of Earth and her creatures. The rich pantheon of deities—kind or evil, mischievous or loving, male and female—these all became abominations.

Earth with her creatures and delicately balanced systems was cast down. The nurturing, supporting entities of antiquity were transformed into enemies, destroyed and despoiled in God's name. If we were good, obedient, servile, the mysterious mind/spirit would be sent into an imagined heaven; our bodies, vile and sinful, condemned to Earth. The old stories became heresies, the life-giving qualities of women were demeaned, love between men and women regulated and restrained. Babies were deemed unclean, born of sin.

As our connection with Earth changed from intimacy to fear and competition, we learned in the new western tradition to disconnect ourselves from our nurturing Earth, to separate our minds and spirits from our bodies. This must have been far more difficult for women than men, as we are traditionally the caregivers and healers of our cultures, comforting those engaged in the life processes of childbirth, growth, illness, death. In a way women have always resisted the split, even when we were ridiculed for our "women's intuition."

Mind and body—intuition and abstract thought—remained separate even into our times. Reluctantly science, the new deity, began to take steps toward greater understanding of the human brain with its two halves. Eventually researchers came to see that each half performed tasks but in different ways. They even cut apart the two hemispheres to "cure" certain mental diseases, well into our century. More recently scientists have concluded that the two halves of the brain work together with the whole body to create a healthy, functioning human being. It has been long in coming and often inhibits us from recognizing the interdependence of mind and body.

Decades ago I tried to keep a dip pen from spluttering ink across a rough, lined tablet, impatient to write down the ideas that pressed so urgently inside my ten-year-old head. I yearned to use my dad's rickety old typewriter. Technology, it seemed, was always better at co-ordinating mind and fingers. I didn't imagine that someday I would be writing on a contraption as magical as a computer. I'm dismayed to find this superb instrument stumbles and hangs up on the same problems as the pen nibs half a century ago—my impatient mind.

Sometimes I'm angry enough at this mechanical magician to threaten its impersonal, dull gray exterior. Or just give up, and sharpen a raven feather into a quill pen, and to hell with progress.

The computer has efficiency but no wisdom, nor can it think my thoughts. Progress in a multisensory society requires more than computers.

Each little set of words goes into a "file" which must be named, and put where it can be found. The computer keeps track of what may encompass the wisdom of the world as so many bytes, not caring at all what they say or where you put them. There are 20 million bytes where I can lose stuff! The machine won't even let me look at it unless I say exactly what I want to see. Files have been known to vanish, never to be seen again. As long as I have *my* act together, and the power is on, the machine will do its thing. When I'm confused or mixed up it just sits and bleeps at me. It doesn't have a mind; it has patterns to follow and those patterns can go on and on forever, repeating the same mistake.

Every now and then the computer splurps up a funny sound and writes "Disk full error" across the screen. Whereupon it refuses to continue writing, no matter how brilliant my line of thought. It means I must change my pathway for it to do what *I* want to do.

Most of our institutions are suffering a disk full error. Some things have just run on too long. To get on with what we know should be done, the disk must be cleared of old documents, outdated copy. Files that no longer apply to the reality of our lives must be searched out and deleted to make room for better data. We need mind and body working at peak efficiency to do it!

Early computerese philosophized, "Garbage In; Garbage Out." I don't hear that very often any more, but it is unclear whether that's because there isn't as much garbage going in, or we have become so accustomed to garbage that we don't notice any more.

Living creatures are not computers, but in some ways our bodies resemble these magical machines. From the heritage of eons bodies know how to live, how to grow, how to keep the systems functioning and the programs running. Unlike the computer, bodies have built-in repair services to mend a thousand tiny flaws. Living things are programmed for maximum wellness, and our personal repair kits are miraculous. We live in a constant state of renewal. Red blood cells are replaced every three days. Brain cells take a longer time to build but they too change and are ready for new programming on a continuing basis. The entire body is said to be replaced every six to seven years. I'm coming up on my eleventh retread. I expect it will be the best model so far. (It doesn't have quite the speed of earlier models, but it works well, and is bigger!)

Besides regenerating itself, the body/mind knows how to regulate blood pressure, exchange oxygen, metabolize food. It also forms thoughts and words to transfer ideas, express our needs and carry on the business of living and loving. A rapidly growing literature confirms that our minds determine *how* the body will respond. As the World Health Organization puts it, good health is *"not merely the absence of disease, but a positive state of physical and mental well-being."*

I have a haunting feeling that the ordinary person's access to her or his own well-being has reached a different level. We forget that we are meant to be healthy. With every twinge of pain, moment of despair, or malfunction we are conditioned to expect illness, and head for doctors. We take their medicines, undergo their operations and expect them to cure us. Often we do this without taking an informed look at the garbage we put in, or accepting the responsibility for clearing out the old files. In seeking healing we should be aware of the power of the mind to make the body sick, and its equally powerful ability to make it well again.

Let me tell you a true story.

Twenty-two years ago in the heart of a big city, a fifty-year-old woman lived in a grand house with every convenience. She had everything anyone could want. Her distinguished husband rose very early in the morning, ate breakfast on the way to work and made plenty of money. She slept in, hated getting up even to dress in her nice clothes. She was miserable. Her back ached so badly she could hardly walk. Except for the days the cleaning woman came, she had to shame herself into getting dressed. What difference does it make? she would ask herself.

She had scarcely enough energy to perform her one daily task—preparing the evening meal on time. Walking three blocks to the corner grocery store was agonizing. It was impossible to drive through chaotic traffic. She had frequent headaches and a listlessness that left her exhausted from a telephone call. Friends rarely came around, and she couldn't go out. Frightening irregular heartbeats took over at any time, sometimes lasting for several hours. Always there was backache. Her children were all away from home, her husband busy with important work.

Sometimes she thought she was dying. It seemed like a good idea, dying. There were several kinds of drugs around the house that would do the job. She looked up doses in a big medical book and knew how much to take and what wouldn't hurt too much. It would be a great relief to get it over with. Her husband said she was a hypochondriac or it was just her "change of life." She was miserable and very depressed.

Finally, a good neighbor took her to a Well Woman's Clinic and checked her in under her maiden name. Just to see. There she was weighed, tested, catheterized, biopsied, prodded, palpated, X-rayed, and CAT-scanned. Blood was withdrawn, urine taken, basal metabolism assessed, endurance measured on a treadmill, and the ordinary things like blood pressure, throat, ears, eyes, anus, breasts, cervix—all examined. The doctors and technicians were very thorough. No part of her body was overlooked or ignored. She was asked no questions and left the clinic after eight hours, miserable and exhausted.

Her follow-up appointment was one week later. By then the samples of her body parts, their fluids and their pictures had been analyzed with the most elaborate machines and the latest medical alchemy. Timidly she returned for the verdict.

"Young lady," the doctor said. They often call women "young

lady" when they have bad news. And he read off strings of results which she understood hardly at all. "That's the good news, and it is good. You also show reduced adrenal tissue and resorption of renal tissue which will lead in due time to blah, blah . . . There are some conservative treatments we can try, but eventually you should consider a transplant—although it doesn't make much sense to have a transplant at your age."

"Am I going to die?" she asked wildly.

"Not soon," he said kindly. "The treatment we will give you will maintain you for some time, and should keep you from feeling any worse."

"That isn't good enough!" she cried bitterly. "I don't want to feel the way I feel. I hate it. Make me well!"

"Don't get hysterical. We can only do the best we can with the very latest equipment and most up-to-date procedures." He named the procedures. "At your age, you must accept that your condition is certain to deteriorate. What would you expect? There, there! Don't cry. You have ten good years ahead of you! Now run along, and make an appointment. Nurse will help you."

"Ten years!" she shrieked. "Ten years!" Suddenly it didn't seem very long. And she returned to the fine big house and cried and cried and wailed, "Why me?" and forgot to get the dinner. She began to sink into a profound depression.

She tried to tell her husband what the doctor had said, but he was so annoyed about dinner not being ready that she didn't tell him anything. He said she'd made him late for his meeting. She didn't even tell him she'd been to the clinic. So she got some sort of dinner together and he went off to his important meeting. Alone again in her lovely house she began to think . . . only ten years left! It's so unfair . . . how can they be "good" years when I feel so rotten . . . I hate this stupid life! I'd rather die than be an invalid! *In-valid*, she thought. Who's to say I'm not valid? No one is in-valid. He did say ten good years. *I've* never had ten good years, all the years have belonged to other people. If these are my years, I'm going to live them my way! That's enough time to do *something for myself!*

So she set out to live for herself. She refused the medical treatment, refused an X-ray course because she felt there had been plenty of X-rays over her lifetime, and they probably didn't do anything more than satisfy curiosity, and might make that damaged kidney act up.

She started doing yoga with the lady on television. The same neighbor who had suggested the clinic also told her about the yoga. She'd never tried it, she felt so rotten, and besides it was some kind of foreign thing. But she tried now, carefully, and felt better and became more flexible day by day. She began to eat good food at lunch and breakfast. What the hell, she thought to herself, I raised three strong, healthy kids. I'm going to do the same for me! And she took lots of vitamin C and went for walks when the weather was fine. And always got the dinner on time. And counted the days of the ten years.

Then one day she asked herself, What, of all the things in the world I've wondered about, would I most like to do? She thought and thought as she walked farther and farther each day. Spring was coming. She began to notice people passing by and see growing things. She found a battered old tree in a park, and noticed it many times. One day, scarred and twisted as it was, it bloomed the length of one small branch—just for her. She put her arms around the tree and cried tears of gratitude. She began to believe anything was possible.

She thought about what she wanted to do, and how it could be done. She woke every morning, her head racing with ideas. She was filled with curiosity, wonder and questions about things she'd rarely thought about in recent years. After some weeks she forgot how rotten she felt, or how much of the ten years was left.

Before long her plan had formed. She was feeling much better. She told her husband, and he said, "Yes, dear," and he went off to a meeting. With $412 in her purse she left the grand house, heading west on the bus with her sterling silver, six small Inuit carvings which she might turn into cash—and a dream.

She found a job paying $100 a week. She lived and worked in rooms rented inexpensively from a friend for whom she had done some favors. She simplified her needs, scaled down her expenses, eventually got a grant, hired some young people, laughed a lot, discovered ingenious ways to expand the dream, found new helpful friends, worried from time to time, learned how to do things she didn't even know existed before, and worked very hard to perfect the dream for ten years. Then the grants ran out.

One day she remembered that ten years was supposed to be zero time. Maybe it had all collapsed because she was going to die. But it wasn't that way at all. It just happened to be the time when she couldn't get any more money to fund the dream. The ghost of the old depression began to taunt her. It was time to make more changes. Once again she packed up her life, headed west. She followed her bliss to a beautiful place by the sea amid tall trees and waves of wildflowers. She has learned to work on a computer, has about $150 a week to live on, and knows that dying, when it comes, will be yet another, even more mysterious stage of the journey. She feels great and is learning to look inside herself. She has discovered that she is old and smart, and that it is just fine.

That's a long story. A poor thing, perhaps, but not bad for someone who was supposed to have been dead for twelve years. What is most remarkable is that I've never felt better in my life.

The story illustrates mind over matter. Sometimes we can decide to heal ourselves. We have a choice about how we feel. Jesse Jackson, the African American activist, said you may not have chosen to be down, but you have a choice as to whether you try to get up. I had a choice all along, but wasn't wise enough to know it. Instead of living in health, I nearly killed myself holding in the bottled-up pain of years.

In his books *Love Medicine & Miracles* and *Peace, Love and Healing,*

Dr. Bernie Siegel says that if we change our state of mind, we may be able to change the course of our illness. He encourages patients to combine establishment medicine with such mind-altering techniques as visualization, meditation, hypnosis—and perhaps the most healing modes of all: love, peace and forgiveness. I would also add hope, for hope is an avenue to the future. Unlike physicians who focus on illness, Dr. Siegel studies *success*. He wonders why one worker exposed to asbestos or radiation comes down with a life-threatening illness while another, equally exposed, manages to avoid it. The reason, he says, is that those who stay well are mentally healthier.

From my observations while working in hospitals, I noticed that cancer patients differ from heart patients in how they show emotion and aggressiveness. Heart patients often seem to be angry, furiously complaining and raising their blood pressure to a point the heart can no longer endure, even to the point of stroke. They tend to be Type-A people. Cancer patients, on the other hand, are usually the "nice" people who rarely complain, trying to do everything everybody wants them to do. They hold so much disappointment and frustration inside that it begins literally to eat up the organs that hold on to their stress.

We need to ask what our illness does for us. Why do we cling to sickness? I'd always tried to be as good as I could be, and spent years of half-life hoping someone would notice, respect my ideas, put me somewhere on their list and show me love. I needed a profound jolt to help me realize that *I* create my health. Only I can pay attention to my needs, my body. No one else will, or can, do it for me. It is so easy to surrender in a downward spiral of misery, and do nothing because one is too distraught to act constructively or too hurt to take charge. Many times when I've felt sorry for myself I've had to ask sternly, "Do you want to be pitied, or do you want to be treated as a worthwhile person?"

What remains most daunting of all is that old phantom, the inability to feel self-love. From talking to many Age Mates, it is clear to me that the ability to put one's self first has been conditioned out of many women of our generation. It was a terrible sin to think well of ourselves, to be proud of our accomplishments, or to feel pretty, when pretty was the only worthwhile thing to be. Nor was it popular with the other kids to be smart in school.

Parents often sneered, "Who do you think you are?" This was soon followed by husbands asking, "What more do you want?" A lifetime spent in our love/service profession has often required us to dismiss our sense of worthiness, to put others first regardless of our own needs.

We would have performed our love/service better, had we the courage to be true to ourselves. Self-love or self-confidence is not conceit. Nor is it ever the rigidity of self-righteousness. Respect for one's own being as a worthy member of creation is essential. One has the right to be, simply because one is alive. "Be here now" is what the hippie children tried to tell us. "And therefore choose life," is another version. "But harm none, do what you will," is the Wiccan philosophy.

Each living person has the right—perhaps even the responsibility—to believe fully, creatively, joyously in his or her own worthiness. It's a mistake to let sickness or self-doubt get in the way of our intriguing possibilities. We can't even guess at what we can become. Having lost my way to the point of creating a life-threatening condition, I intend to stay well. I surely don't want to miss this part of the trip.

When I am overwhelmed by self-doubts, I play this song, now on a tape called *You Are More: Songs of the Possible Human.* It was given to me by my friend, Howard Jerome. The words are worth considering carefully.

You Are More

You are more than you pretend to be
You are more than what most eyes can see
You are more than all your history
Look inside and you will find
There is glory in your mind
Come be the kind of person you could be

You are more than what your leaders say
You are more than how you earn your pay
You are more than what you seem today
So drop that loser's mask
You're equal to the task
The question you should ask is who you are

You are more than some statistic chart
You are more than the sum of all your parts
You are more inside your heart of hearts
You know that it is true
This body that is you
Has miracles to do. Believe!

You are more than what the preachers shout
You are more, come let your spirit out
You are more your soul shall have no doubt
Arise, become awake
With every breath you take
The god within will ache to be.

You are more than cell and blood and bone
You are more than just your name alone
You are more than all that you may own
Look around you everywhere
There is something that we share
The magic in the air is you.

You are more than what your parents bred
You are more than what your teachers said
You are more than what's inside your head
Let your vision now expand, and everybody stand
Come take your neighbour's hand and sing . . .

You are more than you pretend to be
You are more than what most eyes can see
You are more than all your history
Look inside and you will find
That's glory in your mind
You can be the kind of human you can be!
—Howard Jerome and Jean Houston

We are all disoriented to some extent by the profound transformations we are experiencing in these times. A new world attitude is trying to be born. In part, this is related to our science which sees only the surface of things—how many, how much, how big, but not what is within, where it is connected or what it can do. Science did its job very well, but it does not do the whole job, the one required in our changing world.

We see chaos nearly everywhere we look; the solid base of families, religions and governments is falling apart. Along with the confusion, something else is happening that is both enigmatic and quickening. It appears to be developing in and around the human potential movement. Millions are seeing their lives and their world differently.

Look about and see. Search for your way into it. We are engaged in a journey of discovery. Earth herself is saying, "Notice me! See my miracles. Honor me!" Colors seem brighter, flowers more abundant. Maybe the thinning ozone accounts for the changes but it may be far more profound. New ideas and information from the experience of people around the world are coming to our attention. New values are emerging amid all the turmoil.

There are myriad pathways to reach the inner self. It may be that nothing happens by chance, including encounters with kindred spirits. A deeper spirituality is developing. I can't tell what it is, but it points toward a new tomorrow available to souls reaching out to find new ways of being. Even with the clash of cultures seen in many parts of the world, humanity may be approaching the moment when might will not be considered right.

Certain people with certain kinds of genes, personality, exposure to sickness-producing circumstances, contract fatal illnesses. Others with similar backgrounds and environments don't even get sick. Think of Mother Teresa treating lepers for all these years, but not contracting leprosy. Instead of the old put-down, "You made your bed, now lie in it," we could heed the kinder admonition, "Pick up your bed and walk," acknowledging the strength of the spirit, the power of the will, and the astonishing capacity of the body to heal itself. And above all, the power of the mind to profoundly influence that healing. In this emerging era it is important that each of us be strong.

We have been conditioned to blame ourselves for our shortcomings and even for our own illness, to accept the verdict of authority figures and, crudely stated, "to shut up and take it." Sometimes we do make ourselves ill, and even choose particular kinds of diseases that will garner sympathy, attention or a show of meaningful affection. It seems better to take refuge in illness than to be alone so we go to doctors who are often the only persons in whom society will permit us to confide. But we can create our own miracles, working with our own strength, our power of mind over matter, our love and acceptance of ourselves. Those inner qualities may be hard to latch on to, but they are there, waiting. We may be cured from outside; ultimately we can only heal from within.

Hanging on to fears and angers, hates, hurts, and painful memories can make us sick. But if we agree to love ourselves, it is all right to get angry about things that happen to us now. What is so devastating is to carry anger about things that happened yesterday or during childhood. Everyone has a stock of painful memories, rejection, disappointment, ridicule, sorrows over what might have been. They hurt. But we have a choice about whether we forgive others, including our parents, and heal ourselves or let the hurts go on festering.

Let go of negative feelings. The gripes from the past are passed. We can't change them, and holding on may prevent us from taking a brighter turn in the life we live today. It's like weeds in the garden. There's nothing wrong with weeds, except the plants we want to bloom can't flourish when unwanted plants take up the water and nutrients. The negatives that flood through our consciousness consume a lot of energy—the way outdated files in the computer consume megabytes of memory. When negative thoughts and feelings persist they cause ulcers, frown lines, fatigue, weight loss (or gain), bad temper, aches and pains, indigestion, headaches and so on. Hate can kill. Our thoughts are so much a part of everything we do that soothing the mind eases the body and mends the aching heart.

There aren't enough pills in the world to cure *Negativity, Anger and Bitterness*. We have to NAB them whenever they rise up to haunt us. Just grab the thought as it swirls by, and throw the junk out.

Mind-deadening tranquilizers, body-numbing drugs, booze, eating binges, and cigarettes all do something about the angst, but they neither heal nor cure. I have to confess I've tried them all and so have a lot of Age Mates. The only way we will truly feel better is to lighten up. This calls for changes in attitudes, habits, lifestyle, exercise and exercises, devices or mnemonics to help us abandon the old destructive patterns. Stop the negatives dead the moment you feel them rising. Should these persist and become uncontrollable, do seek help from professionals. Obsessions are to be avoided.

Getting rid of these haunting angers has to do with beauty and a good night's sleep. Don't take your angers to bed. NAB them on the spot. Just as you go to sleep, gather pleasant thoughts together—about colors or places or your star, whatever gives you peace. Get comfortable on one side or the other, and as you go to sleep, lock in pleasant thoughts. Say to yourself, "I am a wonderful woman." Place a thumb or finger gently over the frown lines above the bridge of the nose as sleep comes. Keep the love in, including self-love. In all probability, frown lines will begin to fade in a few weeks, and sleep will be more restful.

Frowns accumulate in the area above the pineal gland, near the center of your forehead. The true function of that mysterious gland is imperfectly understood. Certain animals are thought to sense light or direction through it. Some cultures attach great importance to this area. It is the site of the Third Eye, known throughout world folklore. It is where Hindu women and holy men place the *bindi*. It is where the Cyclops has his eye, where David hit Goliath and where we gather our tension into frown lines. I suspect the pineal gland has a species-deep meaning for living things, which we don't yet understand. Perhaps, if we establish the space above the pineal body as a still center, other parts of our lives will flow more harmoniously.

The promo on the back of Shakti Gawain's powerful little book, *Creative Visualization*, makes a remarkable claim: "An introduction to the art of using mental energy to transform and greatly improve health, beauty, prosperity, loving relationships, and the fulfillment of all your desires."

Creative visualization is a system in which you use imagination to create your life the way you want it to be and to get rid of things you do not want. You just think up—*image*—what you desire, get it very clear in your mind, focus on your goal from time to time, and through some remarkable combination of qualities within yourself and in the universe, changes will come. The changes may not be exactly what you expect, but you will feel very good about them.

You need no tools, no totems, no hard-to-find tapes—only imagination with which you create a clear image of something you wish to happen.

Perhaps you have heard about the technique of imagining healthy white blood cells surrounding diseased cells in the body and consuming them. In more and more places visualization is used with conventional medicine to hasten the cure of everything from leukemia to broken bones. One imagines the physical situation as it should be, whole and functioning and in good health, then focuses the mind on the body's natural defenses, bringing them to bear on the problem. After a while, the condition improves. A person with a damaged spine focuses on how it feels to walk, repeats it time and again, believes that she will walk, and tries. In due course new nerve pathways are established, and she walks! Of course it will not work completely in all cases, nothing does, but improvements happen often enough to make it worthwhile to explore the healing possibilities of one's inner strengths before undergoing more invasive procedures. It is much better than giving in to sickness or giving up.

The healing comes from within the body itself. When we regularly allow ourselves quiet and inner peace we no longer need to get sick in order for our inner self to get attention.

If creative visualization interests you, I urge you to buy Shakti's book. I know no other investment that will open grander avenues to explore. I wish it had been available years ago through many of my traumas. What mechanisms are actually at work, I do not know, but I believe it is part of Creation's intention that we receive wellness from the powers of life.

One of the exercises described is called "Creating Your Sanctuary." It is one of the first things to try, and will serve you long and happily. A number of women I've talked to report that they have tried the technique successfully. The sanctuary is within yourself—some imagined place for your mind to go where you feel safe, protected, at peace. Shakti describes the process this way:

> Close your eyes and relax in a comfortable position. Imagine yourself in some beautiful natural environment. It can be any place that appeals to you . . . in a meadow, on a mountaintop, in the forest, beside the sea . . . even on another planet. Wherever it is, it should feel comfortable, pleasant and peaceful to you. Explore your environment, noticing the visual details, the sounds and smells, any particular impressions you get about it.
>
> Now do anything you would like to make the place more homelike and comfortable for you. You may want to build some type of house or shelter there, or perhaps just surround the whole area with a golden light of protection and safety, create and arrange things there for your convenience and enjoyment, or do a ritual to establish it as your special place. From now on this is your own personal inner sanctuary, to which you can return at any time just by closing your eyes and desiring to be there. You will always find it healing and relaxing. It is also a place of special power for you. . . . Your sanctuary may change from time to time, or you may want to make changes. . . . Just remember to retain the primary qualities of peacefulness, tranquility and a feeling of absolute safety.

I was desperately homesick during the war years, yearning for my Oregon home. There was nobody who knew its special beauty or what it meant to me. The people in that Eastern city had it in their heads that everyone from "the West" was some sort of ignorant hick who rode a horse to school, and punched cattle, whatever that meant.

So I built Oregon in my mind's eye, a place to dream in and feel at home. That was long before I knew such imaginings had a name. My Place, which was all I ever called it, was in a meadow of wildflowers by water. A snug little house with lots of windows stood in the center. Great evergreens encircled the meadow, their straight, tall trunks creating tranquility and peace. Wild flowers bloomed, waves lapped softly on the beach. Different kinds of birds chirped and sang. I could have seagulls and eagles fly over the water. Every now and then a deer wandered into my make-believe meadow. I came and went as my need decreed, often falling to sleep "listening" to the gentle waves. My Place probably kept me sane during those difficult years and has comforted me ever since.

And now for something completely amazing! The above is a nearly perfect description of the place I live right now! Is it possible that I imagined it into being? Did it materialize out of nowhere to become available to me and give such joy and security?

When I first came here, the move was fraught with many complications—things like mortgages, shortages of money and water, and a roof that leaked when it finally rained. I didn't exactly "see" where I was. A year or so later, just as the curly lilies were in bloom, my mind swung in a dizzying circle and I was back in my Oregon dream, only I was in *this* beloved place. Did wishing make it so?

May your visualizations be as fruitful, and as comforting.

How often does your head surge with torrents of words? Unending chatter coming unbidden from every direction? Nearly everyone finds these imaginary discussions going on. Sometimes it's depressing just listening in. The chit-chat usually has nothing to do with the moment at hand, and often makes concentration difficult. Conversations may range from arguments with long-gone relatives to the perfect squelch for a cheeky check-out person. Rafts of "I wish I'd said" appear on our screens. Often the sheer volume of mental traffic clouds our ability to deal meaningfully with whatever needs attention. There seems no end to words dredged up from the depths, hauled in from afar, or writ on distant clouds of memory.

Stress comes from various causes—responsibility, grief, tension, overwork, unhappiness. When it builds up, it profoundly affects the processes in our bodies. Blood pressure rises, the immune system tightens up, nerves are on edge and the mind is a jungle of static. But we need a clear mind/body and brain to function most effectively, especially when we are under a great deal of stress.

Meditation can produce the needed state of tranquility. It has been called the healing silence.

Most of us have heard about it. Many of our children, mine included, discovered meditation in their wandering years. Transcendental Meditation (TM) was introduced into North America in the 1960s with claims for peace and understanding that were startling. In the non-Western world, meditation has been practiced for centuries by millions of people. It is based on a Vedic tradition originating thousands of years ago in the Far East.

As with most non-technical ideas, our culture viewed TM with suspicion. Several professions felt threatened by the invasion of such "foreign" influences, and set to work to denounce or discredit it. During the intervening years meditation has been through the fine comb of scientific scrutiny—probed, prodded and measured by skeptical researchers. They did hundreds of double-blind studies, made comparisons, wired yogis and other meditators with heart, blood pressure, temperature and immune response machines.

The practice of meditation was found to be legitimate! Just as the Maharishi said, meditation soothes the mind, relaxes the body and creates a feeling of peace. Herbert Benson, a Harvard cardiologist, calls this the relaxation response (RR). His 1975 book by that name was a best seller. Benson discovered that all major religious traditions use simple, repetitive prayers very like meditation. Such repetitions create RR, the exact opposite to stress reactions.

Without apparent exception, Western medicine has found no

harm in meditation. Meditation is now thought to have a positive effect on the individual's sense of well-being. Used in conjunction with other therapies, meditation enhances conventional treatment of certain serious diseases.

It is effective in calming the heart and reducing blood pressure. An even more dramatic discovery is the ability of meditators to influence their immune systems. The mind can actually call forth a range of disease-fighting mechanisms from within the body and relieve symptoms.

Meditation is free and can be practiced anywhere, as I learned some years ago in Japan. A woman I didn't know, walking just ahead of me on a busy Tokyo street, clearly demonstrated the adaptability of meditation and/or prayer. Hundreds of people were rushing along the sidewalk which passed one of the many Shinto shrines dotting Japanese cities. Without preliminaries the woman stopped, bowed her head, clapped her hands three times, and was utterly apart from the hurrying throng. I almost bumped into her. The crowd flowed around her. She stood alone, head bowed, unperturbed among hundreds. My companion, answering my unspoken query, said the woman was communing with her ancestors. The passing crowd, it seemed, understood and respected her need.

Once the technique is learned, meditation becomes an effective, personal, fully portable "energizer" to be used wherever you are. You *can't* leave home without it. It costs nothing and helps us achieve control over our lives, which may be why it isn't more widely prescribed. Not only do meditators feel better, they also look better, appear less harried and more alive. Michael Toomey and colleagues at Britain's Meru Research Institute found that meditators scored an average seven years younger than their actual ages when they were tested for hearing, visual acuity and systolic blood pressure. Further research confirmed the longer a person has been meditating, the more age-resistant he or she is. It is a simple enough principle, but a powerful one. As muscles relax, the mind quiets down and sagging spirits revive. We are more able to take charge of our lives. *And* we look better!

There are many levels of and numerous refinements to the practice of meditation. We did it instinctively as children lost in thought. It isn't relearned all at once, but even a beginning effort will show results if you want it to. I was initially put off by the myth that one needed a kind of initiation to qualify for a "mantra" (this turns out not to be essential), and I couldn't achieve the "lotus" position without discomfort. The real truth is I was afraid of what I would find by looking into my inner self. (It turns out there was nothing *too* scary inside.)

Acquiring the ability to meditate may be difficult for women. In our busy years we customarily do several things at once. You know the sequence—dialing the plumber while deciding on what to make for dinner, listening to the kids play out back where you really should bring in the laundry before you leave for the grocery store and you trust there's enough gas. "Hello, Joe's Plumbing?"

Women's lives include numerous layers of responsibility. It may be one of the unacknowledged differences between the sexes. It seems men focus on one thing, attempting to reach it in a straight line. If women did that the kids would fall out of the tree. But most Age Mates have time now to try getting through the thought layers to explore the world with a meditator's clear, untroubled mind. You'll find it interesting, even rewarding.

To begin an exploration of the benefits of meditation there are three things to keep in mind: posture, breath and attitude in the *now*. Past, present and future do not figure in meditation. I have begun to practice meditation before each day's writing session. It has been helpful, especially in focusing my thoughts, and helps me keep writing for six or seven hours each day.

It takes a few minutes to tune out the hundreds of daily concerns and focus my attention on breathing. To "tune in" to that inner self, just shove intruding thoughts gently away.

In brief, this is the process: Find a quiet, comfortable place. Unplug the phone so you can have your time undisturbed. If you are agile, sit cross-legged on the floor, but most Age Mates find a chair with a straight back more comfortable. The purpose is to have your spinal column straight. Place your feet flat on the floor, your hands relaxed in your lap, palms up as a gesture of receptivity. Set yourself the length of time you plan to sit, and stick with it. Ten minutes will do in the beginning. Twenty minutes is the time TM suggests, but that's after some practice.

To begin close your eyes. Take three *slow*, deep breaths and allow yourself to relax completely. Breathe from the diaphragm, pushing out the stomach on inhalation, pushing it in to exhale. Let go of the concerns and cares of the moment. (When they come to mind, tell them to go away, you will deal with them later. This is *your* time to be totally focused within yourself.) Inwardly state your intentions ("I choose to refresh myself in this still time") or say a short prayer.

Take another deep breath. Exhale slowly. Allow the next inhalation to emerge naturally, automatically, from inside you. Focus your attention on this breath and ride it like a wave. Feel the breath flowing inside you, from deep in your abdomen to your nostrils, and back down.

Count "one" on the inhale, "two" on the exhale, "three" on the next inhalation, and so on to ten, then start again. Allow each numbered breath to fill your mind.

When thoughts wander, return your mind to the count and begin again with one. Don't be angry at yourself, just start over. Don't search for insights, phenomena or communication. Simply *be*. Keep *being* until the time is up. It passes rapidly.

Close your meditation by imagining yourself surrounded by a sphere of golden light, and thank the Higher Powers. In the beginning do not be concerned so much with the actual length of time, as long as you make some moments to meditate every day, preferably near the same time and in the same place. You will automatically go into a meditative state as you start your day or approach the task before you.

For variations, meditate on a lighted candle, a flower, a feather, a crystal or an unusual stone. Or go outside and find a special tree, a stream or clouds. Contemplate this natural object *without thought* for fifteen minutes or more. Simply observe it. This is a powerful means of connecting with the Earth, entrusting your mind to Nature's miraculous care. Fix upon a word to repeat with each breath. Allow it to become your mantra. As your spirit soars, thank the Earth for her bounty.

As our minds gradually still, life itself becomes more tranquil and clear. We begin to see into the depths of our inner spirits, allowing our own light to emerge.

Dr. Benson's research found that people who use prayers rather than mere phrases stay with the method longer. He then worked with religious researchers on a related phenomenon he calls the Faith Factor. He suggests that the benefits of faith may interact with the direct physiological benefits of RR and that prayer sets up the interaction.

People high in spirituality—which Benson defines as the feeling that "there is more than just you" and is not necessarily religious—scored high in physiological health. They had fewer stress-related symptoms. Next he found that people high in spirituality gain the most from meditation training. They show the greatest rise on a "life-purpose index" as well as the sharpest drop in pain.

The spiritual leaders—from religious sociologists to monastic orders to rabbis—who participated in the meditation/prayer exploration became more convinced that prayer seems to do some of the things they'd always hoped, and maybe a lot more. Prayer together with meditation strengthened the spirit, calmed the mind and healed the body.

After centuries of offering misplaced guidance, the learned ones— theologians as well as scientists—may be ready to ask deep questions. Maybe they will look for qualities of healing as well as treatments.

As environmental consciousness dawns widely, we may be able to return to the once-sacred notion of healthy humans in a healthy place. To do this we have our multisensory consciousness to call upon. As the spiritual attributes of individuals, political systems, and the interdependence of life on Earth are recognized, we will make it safe to value common sense. Common sense is a step toward healing. It can help us discern what is wise and what is false. Since women generally do not have, and are not conditioned to covet, the power to suppress others, we know the difference between right and wrong in our own hearts. Let us have the courage to use our common sense, and act accordingly. Women's intuition includes the ability to make sensible decisions. There have been more than enough "studies" by experts and far too many excuses for continuing unwise practices.

> North America has gone from naive to jaded without ever passing wise. —Author unknown

There is so much that needs healing, beginning with how we think about ourselves and our surroundings. We are such a cerebral lot, choosing to overlook what we do not wish to see. The changes during our lifetimes—technological, social, political, economic, medical—have taken place with scant regard for consequences.

Dazzled by the brilliance of thoughtless genius, we willy-nilly do anything and everything that can be done whether it means destroying ecosystems, damming rivers, eroding topsoil, exterminating species—as long as it can be done for profit. Too often we simply opt out of decision-making and let the tide sweep us down the polluted beach. The time has arrived to play Truth or Consequences for keeps! It is time for women to consult our common sense and our best life-creating, culture-giving instincts, and to insist our men and boys do what is right. Just as the mind is not separate from the body, Earth is not separate from her human occupants nor is her future independent from our efforts to heal. We need to put our minds to it!

CHAPTER 9

THE CARE AND TREATMENT OF DOCTORS

Some of our best friends are doctors, but we must stand on guard for our own well-being. The health needs of older women are poorly understood. Treatment is often inappropriate, sometimes even harmful. This is disheartening since the medical profession often seems to be the only culturally acceptable place to tell our troubles.

We are conditioned to look upon doctors as lesser deities. Our very sense of security is threatened when we are cautioned to be on guard against fallibility in the profession we have trusted and venerated for a lifetime.

It seems older women are not particularly well liked by the medical profession. A blatant double standard exists for the way men and women are treated. According to no less an authority than the United States Public Health Service Task Force on Women's Health Issues (May 1985), women are treated with less respect within the health care system, and receive poorer medical care than men. Older women face double jeopardy. The overwhelming majority of doctors in North America are male. The illnesses of women, especially "old" women, are seen to be of less importance, and prevention is often not deemed worth the time it takes the doctor to explain. Men are deemed to have "real" illness; women are regarded as neurotic and troublesome, and old women hardly worth treating. With the high costs of medical care and the financial drain on individuals, surely change is called for!

The consideration and concern shown older male patients recovering from prostectomy, as a case in point, is almost laughable. An instruction sheet (given to the wife) spells out proper home care. It states, among other things: no driving or riding for three weeks!—levitation home from the hospital, no doubt—no heavy work like raking leaves or taking out the garbage, no intercourse for two months, and so on. Compare that to a woman who has just given birth, and whose reproductive organs have also been worked over. In my time, she was expected to return home in five or six days, nurse the infant, care for the other children, get dinner that night, and be available for sexual activity after six weeks. Who ever thought taking out the garbage had anything to do with heavy work? Today many new mothers are sent home after twenty-four hours, with minimal attention to their support systems.

Whatever the circumstances, women are seldom welcome to stay in the sick role as long as men are. Because our culture conditions us never to need care unless we are very sick, women must often think up "presenting" symptoms in order to justify consulting a doctor, even though the problem may be more emotional than physical. We are often shunted from one specialist to another with no "cure." This is not a call for more psychiatrists. Aging people, especially women, need help with their changing lives, not their complexes. I am dismayed by how little is known about the physiological changes women undergo during menopause, considering that it is experienced by *half the population*.

Why does the medical profession treat females differently? The definitive explanation will have to come from the practitioners themselves, but we will serve *ourselves* better if we realize there are differences. Knowledge of and control over our bodies is fundamental. We must insist on our right to know how the medical profession treats us as we age, and stop relinquishing our bodies to the control of others.

The general attitude that aging is a disease confuses gerontology—the *study* of aging, with geriatrics—the *treatment* of the aged. Although the aging population is growing rapidly, neither discipline is adequately included in the education of doctors. Eric Sevareid commented in the April 1991 issue of *Modern Maturity* that it is "scandalous that as the older population rapidly increases, the American Medical Association, with a total membership of 290,000, still includes only 586 doctors whose practices concentrate on geriatrics."

Because medicine is male-dominated, both researchers and study subjects in gerontology have considered health problems in the aged as largely male problems, possibly not noticing that women experience aging and illness differently, or that women will live many aged years longer than men. The shortcomings of a patriarchal culture are nowhere more obvious than in the practice of medicine.

Society's attitudes are so deeply rooted, it is possible doctors do not know they discriminate against women. I first encountered prejudice in gross anatomy class, where I saw ludicrous efforts to avoid dissecting a female cadaver. Long ago in my job as lab technician on a cardiovascular research project, I participated in a number of autopsies along with pathologists and student doctors. The experience sickened me, not because of the autopsies, but because of the degrading remarks directed toward female deceased. Whether or not the gross antics were for my benefit is impossible to say, but it was disgusting. Their attitudes must surely have filtered into other aspects of their practice.

Crude jokes were leveled not only at the female bodies but also at female students. Thirty years ago, promising women students, sometimes at the head of the class, dropped out because life was made miserable by the "real" student doctors. My direct experience was with the big eastern US schools in the days when one or two women might be admitted to first-year medicine, but no blacks, and there was a 5 percent quota for Jews because that was their proportion in the population. When asked why women, who are 50 percent of the population, were not proportionately included, the establishment answered to the effect, "Why should medical schools waste time training women when they'll just quit in a few years to have kids?"

The difficulty women encounter in medical school is in contrast to their experience after graduation. While women may still have trouble being accepted in established clinics, once they hang up their shingles, women doctors are quickly booked up. Some of their patients are men, but it is greatly liberating for women patients to be able to discuss physiological problems with another woman whose knowledge comes from experience as well as from a textbook. Age Mates report they feel more open about discussing difficulties and less shy when a female physician examines their bodies. Fortunately for all of us, gender equality in medicine is changing dramatically. Medical schools now generally admit between 20 to 40 percent women as first-year students, but this increase has taken more than a century.

THE RISE OF THE SPECIALIST

Sometime in the last half-century the practice of medicine came to a fork in the road. The path less travelled was that of the personal, hands-on family physician/healer/counselor who believed he had a calling to ensure patient health. The glamour of technology and miraculous pharmacology beckoned along the other path and was followed by the majority of physicians who today situate themselves in office fortresses. Patients go to them, even Age Mates with serious illnesses or disabilities. We seldom see our generation's image of the Rockwell Kent doctor sitting by the patient's bed into the wee hours. If we can't get to the busy doctor's office for consultation, we either stay sick at home or call an ambulance!

There has also been a remarkable degree of specialization since our doctor images were formed. Because so much more knowledge is available, doctors focus on different areas of finely tuned expertise in which their specialty may be practiced with little reference to other parts or functions of the body.

It is a costly fault of the system that doctors refer patients to one specialist after another. One is entitled to wonder if the numerous referrals are a contemporary form of "fee-splitting," a practice outlawed years ago after many scandals. Each referral requires hours of patients' time in offices where as many as twelve appointments are booked for the same hour, not to mention the cost and time of transportation, additional tests, anxiety, and almost always additional drugs.

In 1952 I was taken to hospital with an emergency back problem, and was immediately sent for exploratory X-rays. I was about six weeks pregnant, and begged them not to take X-rays, having read even in those days that X-rays were suspected of damaging the fetus. In words of one syllable I was told obstetrics was not their concern. It was that infant's life that gave me the Near Death Experience described in Chapter 18.

Rather than listening to patients, modern specialists appear to place their trust chiefly in sophisticated laboratory tests and other diagnostic procedures. Sometimes the patient seems to be merely the vehicle by which the ailment reaches the office. This sort of impersonal, mechanical treatment results in fewer "cures," ever-growing medical costs, and questionable medication—not to mention patient anxiety.

HEALTH CARE ALTERNATIVES

The time is at hand for the medical profession to re-evaluate the efficacy and allure of expensive high-tech procedures, exotic pharmaceuticals and ever more minute specializations. The kind of medicine practiced by the American and Canadian Medical Associations is the primary form of health care for less than a third of the world's population.

The emphasis of Western medicine is on trauma and acute conditions, rarely on prevention or the long-term effects of chronic treatment. Health care management, by means other than those which are medically based, is hard to come by, although in some places the situation is changing. So certain is the medical profession of its excellence that various alternate forms of treatment are forbidden or even illegal. This remains true despite the effects of intrusive and frequently fallible procedures conjured up by "modern" medicine.

Seventy percent of all prescription medicines originated from natural plants. (Incidentally, many of them are native to the world's rain forests which our generation is rapidly depleting.) Digitalis from foxglove was used to treat heart disease in Asia long before it was accepted as medicine in this culture. Some American Indian women practiced birth control by chewing stoneseed, an herb that contains an estrogen-like substance. Certain natural molds were used to arrest infections before Western medicine discovered penicillin—in mold. Willow bark and roots are still widely used to reduce fever and soothe sore throats. They contain salicylic acid, which is the main ingredient in the much-patented aspirin. Quinine, from cinchona tree bark, was not satisfactorily synthesized until troops fighting in the Pacific had to be rescued from malaria.

Why should there be continuing resistance to exploring other models of health care in the interest of disease prevention and health maintenance? Medicine *can* change. After all, doctors rarely bleed patients now.

The medical profession protects its privileges and prevents patients from consulting with practitioners outside the protected area. Consultation with practitioners who offer non-medical procedures is discouraged, often ridiculed, and in some areas denied to all but the most persistent. The exclusion of chiropractors is perhaps the most obvious example. When her doctor was on vacation, an Age Mate of fifty-five who had suffered years of severe back pain finally went on her own to a chiropractor and received considerable immediate relief. When her MD returned, he refused to treat her ever again. While it is true there are quacks out there, we shouldn't forget that quacks may also occupy offices whose walls are covered with diplomas.

The late Nobel laureate, Linus Pauling, who I am honored to have counted among my medical friends, wrote in his valuable guide to aging, *How to Live Longer and Feel Better*:

> When it comes to concern about health, an important question is the extent to which a person in the United States should depend on his or her physician. At the present time the main job of the physician is to try to cure the patient when he or she appears in the office with a specific illness. The physician usually does not make any great effort to prevent the illness or to strive to put the person consulting him or her in the best of health.
>
> You will be advised to consult doctors only when you believe that you are truly ill. By restricting your medical encounters to those that are absolutely necessary you will be avoiding the risks inherent in most diagnostic and therapeutic procedures.
>
> This advice tends to slight an important function that doctors have assumed in our society: dealing with patients whose main problem is an unhappy life. It is your privilege

to consult a doctor for that purpose, but you should know that few doctors have high cure rates for unhappy lives, so that the chances of obtaining real help are small. Moreover your visit may start a series of potentially dangerous medical tests and treatments.

If, as a result of reading this book, you see that *even a decision to consult a doctor* is a serious and potentially risky one, that it requires some estimate of potential risks as well as potential benefits, you will have spent your time well.

GET A SECOND OPINION ON SURGERY

Surgery for women appears to be the therapy of choice of many doctors. If the patient is female and unwell, the femaleness must be the cause of the malaise, and it ought to be cut out. Some hospitals and practitioners regard hysterectomies as a routine "preventative" medical practice for women over forty-five! There seems to be little or no consideration given to the sense of loss or mutilation resulting from hysterectomies, nor to the disorientation which follows the cessation of menstrual periods. Surgery denies us the experience of the natural changes our bodies undergo through menopause. Many women feel maimed, less feminine and certainly more confused without the experience of declining menstruation, not to mention complications from hormone therapy.

Each year, 650,000 hysterectomies—roughly one every thirty seconds—are performed in the United States. More than 2,000 women die from the operation and another 240,000 suffer major complications. More women die from hysterectomies than die from uterine or cervical cancer which the procedure is intended to cure. So common is the operation that one in three American women undergo surgical rather than natural menopause. The figure in Canada may be as high as 40 percent in some jurisdictions. "Hacking" preventively is absurd and dangerous.

Menopausal women are not the only victims of surgical enthusiasm. Since the female reproductive process has been medicalized, the motto often seems to be "cure it with a cut." Young women are subjected to births by caesarean section in enormously greater numbers than previous generations without a corresponding decrease in mortality. Busy doctors, many of whom resist the assistance of midwives, often find it too costly to take the time to permit a baby to arrive naturally. I asked one doctor why there were so many C-sections. He told me it was hospital policy not to let a labor go more than eight hours! Surgery is also significantly more lucrative.

In *Small Expectations*, Leah Cohen documents surgical preferences in her chapter "Older Women and Health: The Hazards We Face." Gall bladder problems, for example, are a frequent surgical target, especially if the patient can be described as 4F—fair, fat, female and forty. Be wary of surgery.

No doubt a certain number of radical interventions are life-saving. But the medical profession has an unfortunate tendency to rush into highly invasive procedures. That women have more numerous operations—and more repeat operations—than males prompts several questions.

1. Do women, who naturally live longer than men, really have that many more things go wrong inside of them?
2. How much *does* the medical profession actually know about the way women's bodies work?
3. Why is there such readiness to perform surgery on women, often on a "just in case" basis (e.g. hysterectomy because the uterus *may* become cancerous) compared to the cautious approach to operations on men, often with weeks or months of evaluation?
4. Why are the overwhelming majority of organ transplants

performed on men? Do women have fewer critical organ-destroying ailments?

Surgery takes place in hospitals, and hospitals can be dangerous to your health. They are known to harbor an increasing number of antibiotic-resistant organisms. And they have the power to create "non-people" by taking over the lives of persons who surrender to their care. The institution can ignore individuality, make decisions for patients, limit mobility, enforce conformity, scarcely tolerate suggestions. Why is a patient awakened from a sound sleep at 5:00 a.m. to have her temperature taken? Why is a wash basin of hot water thrust at her so the night nurse can go off shift at 6:00? Who are hospitals supposed to serve? A hospital can be the ultimate control device, where commands are given with bed pans, thermometers and food trays. And nurses should not be placed in the position of treating patients badly because of hospital policies or budget priorities. Dr. Pauling always claimed he was not going to a hospital unless someone carried him!

In *Limits of Medicine: Medical Nemesis*, Ivan Illich states:

> The medical establishment has become a major threat to health. . . . One of every five patients admitted to a typical research hospital acquires an iatrogenic (doctor-caused) disease, sometimes trivial, usually requiring special treatment, and in one case in 30 leading to death. Half of these episodes resulted from the complications of drug therapy; amazingly, one in ten came from diagnostic procedures.

It is unsettling to find the heroic doctor of our dreams shot down in ineptitude. Many, possibly even most, deserve the respect and affection we accord them. But we must remember that our beloved Drs. Kildare, Welby and Arrowsmith are fictional. The real world is different, especially because we older women are definitely not "high prestige" patients. Doctors want to cure things. They may not be able to face the incurability of aging, possibly because they themselves will so soon be subject to its slings and arrows.

We must also remember that the medical profession does a questionable job of regulating itself. Recourse through the courts for patient abuse or malpractice is very costly, and next to impossible to substantiate. Doctors rarely testify against colleagues, and dead patients make poor witnesses.

MEDICATION

We are an over-medicated society, expecting that some kind of wonder drug will cure whatever ails us. Many, many people consuming prescription and nonprescription drugs know next to nothing about the drugs they are taking. The profession has recently made a laudable effort to inform patients in a book produced by the Canadian Medical Association and *Readers Digest*. It can help us understand what drugs do to our bodies, and so help avoid serious health problems, perhaps even premature death. The title is *Guide to Prescription and Over the Counter Drugs*. Ask your library to carry the book in its reference section where it can be consulted by the many who need to know.

Some of the confused and senile among us get to be that way as the direct result of over-medication and the effects of one drug acting on another. An astonishing percentage of hospital admissions are related to medication reactions. The situation is worse in long-term care institutions where the "spaced-out" grandmother, lost in a medicated fog oblivious to her surroundings, is depressingly common. As Linus Pauling wrote, studies exploring what happens when medication is *stopped* show that "the patient is rarely worse and may be much improved."

A friend suffering from the mysterious disease lupus was

confused and in pain. She was being treated by three different doctors and taking nine prescribed medications each day, one of which, I knew from experience, seriously disturbed the nervous system. Once she had access to some published drug reports, she asked the doctors to consult with each other, and then stopped some of the medication on her own. Fortunately the disease went into remission and she is again the bright, talented person I knew.

Adult North America might be said to be on a drug treadmill. This may be as damaging to society as the social drugs favored by the young and restless—both kinds are addicting, and ultimately destructive. The difference is that illegal drugs are profitable to the underworld; licit drugs are profitable for the establishment.

The powerful and well-protected pharmaceutical industry ranks very near the top of all profit-making undertakings, higher even than armaments. It plays upon the vulnerability of individuals, and as aging women become a larger part of the population, legal drugs become ever more lucrative. For example, Valium sells for 140 times its manufacturing costs! In this highly profitable, highly competitive field, drug molecules are manipulated to create "new" drugs, too often with insufficient awareness of side effects. Thalidomide was one such example. Pharmaceuticals of this sort are not made for patients; they are made to compete for the bottom line.

Regulatory bodies tend to grant ready approval to drugs developed through accepted channels. The medical profession is so emphatically partial to either surgery or the "prescription fix" that conservative management through diet, exercise, massage, acupuncture or other non-medical treatments are either denied or disparaged. There's not much prestige or money in the time it takes to counsel senior female patients. It is faster and more profitable to urge drugs on us.

The pharmaceutical industry employs an army of "detail men" to persuade the medical practitioner to prescribe their particular wares and distribute their samples. It also maintains powerful lobbies in legislative centers such as Washington, Ottawa and

London. Some companies are generous with political contributions. Some give grants to hard-pressed universities and researchers. They employ galleries of artists, script writers and public relations people to create seductive advertising. Twenty years ago drug companies spent approximately $5,000 per doctor in advertising. It is no doubt considerably higher now. Given the large number of pharmaceutical compounds coming on the market each year, it is impossible for busy physicians to evaluate the efficacy of each one, and thus they are often obliged to accept the verdict of the detail men.

Addictive mood-altering drugs are a booming business. Clinicians who expect women to suffer from psychosomatic illnesses are likely to overlook serious female illness and to treat women with potentially addicting medication. Women are twice as likely as men to receive prescriptions for mood-altering drugs. Forty-four percent of *all* tranquilizers are prescribed for women over fifty-five. One in five Canadian women is ingesting these compounds by prescription, many more from over-the-counter sales. Thanks to the efforts of pharmaceutical houses in the United States, we have no protection against over-prescription and monopoly control of drug prices, so Canadian expenditures on drugs more than doubled in less than a year. We can no longer choose the less expensive generic drugs, and patients lose another aspect of control while the cost of medical care soars.

Rather than helping prevent illness by appropriate counseling (by nurse practitioners, paramedics, social workers and home care helpers), where women can discuss ways to deal with their fears and anxieties, the medical profession and the drug companies often combine to discourage such practices. Drug ads for the profession are specifically aimed at convincing doctors that men may have real ailments, but women's ailments, being psychosomatic, merit increased pharmaceutical treatment.

It must be said that we contribute to our own over-medication by requesting or even insisting that our doctors administer drugs we have heard about in the popular press. Some of us even "shop around" until we find a doctor who will give them to us.

Consumers of medicines are rarely informed of another important fact, and that is the change in the body itself. Just as bones may become brittle and joints stiffen, other organs may become less efficient. For example, the youthful liver gradually removes drugs from circulation by making them water-soluble for excretion in urine. Older livers are less effective in metabolizing drugs and aging kidneys less efficient in excreting them. This can cause drugs to accumulate and reach dangerous levels in the older body.

Three hundred years ago, the French writer Molière wrote, "Nearly all men die of their medicines, not their diseases." We must maintain constant vigilance to be sure that particular bit of wisdom does not repeat itself indefinitely.

PATIENTS' RIGHTS

The doctor is not God. He probably doesn't want to be God, although he may enjoy the benefits. The first thing to know is that you do not cease to be a thinking individual merely because you present yourself to a doctor or a hospital. You have rights, and although they may not seem important to many in the medical establishment, growing numbers of patients are identifying and insisting on their rights. Preventive medicine is more cost-effective as well. It is infinitely less expensive to help a person feel well in the first place than to keep her or him on the merry-go-round of specialists, diagnostic procedures, medication, surgery and more surgery, and eventually intensive care.

Don't be mystified or beguiled by medical jargon you don't understand. You have a right to complete information on your condition in language you can understand, including the treatment proposed, chances of recovery, how long you are likely to be ill, what side effects you can expect from treatment and what alternate therapies are available. As a patient you have the following rights:

1. Right to consent to or refuse treatment.
2. Right to privacy and confidentiality.
3. Right to be told if you are being used in teaching or experimentation, and the right to refuse such.
4. Right to be treated in an emergency.
5. Right to leave a hospital or doctor's office whenever you decide.
6. Right to consult with other physicians.

Informed consent includes the right to refuse during treatment as well as before treatment, and you must agree voluntarily, without coercion or intimidation from physician, family members or others. You do not have to accept "It is just routine" as an explanation for any treatment.

It is essential to read a consent form with care. One Age Mate I talked to had given such consent and found herself involved in a long and painful series of injections that had little if any relevance to her condition, and was extremely costly. She quite unwittingly discovered she had become part of a drug-testing experiment, and as yet has not totally recovered her health. Take a trusted person with you if you need assistance to read the form, understand its language or ask questions.

The feeling is widespread that the professional colleges have too much autonomy and too little accountability. The number of malpractice suits against the profession has skyrocketed in recent years. So has the cost of insurance to doctors and, accordingly, their fees.

I hope the medical profession will look critically at itself and take steps to remedy the problems that have developed in recent decades. The noble calling of the medical doctor requires far more than an awareness of the bottom line. Doctors, like all of us, must strive to be as good as they can be. Being rich in money or prestige should be secondary.

As the proportion of older people increases, doctors will need more effective instructions in geriatrics. Above all, the medical profession *must* recognize its discriminatory practices against older female patients. We are here now, and millions will follow us.

It is encouraging to both patients and physicians that research into and information about aging is becoming more available. In the two decades between the White House Conferences on Aging, 1961 and 1981, more papers on geriatrics and aging were published than in all medical reporting before then, and the number continues to grow. It is comforting to know that our children will have far better access to knowledge about aging than we enjoy. We can hope that it will apply equally to males and females.

Each of us has the right to die with dignity. Sometimes life's struggles, pain and suffering call for mercy. This is a difficult, touchy matter to be weighed with utmost care. But maybe some of us have lived as long as we want to live. Maybe some of us do not want heroic, high-tech intervention. A patient who dies is not an insult to the doctor; she or he is fulfilling the life cycle. Decisions about when life should end can be reached co-operatively, not only by the almighty physician exercising power over the patient. All most of us want is the opportunity to live well until we die, and to insist on the option to stop when the time has come. Some communities have organized Hemlock Societies to advise patients of their rights and choices. I urge you to contact such organizations at an appropriate time.

A Letter to My Doctor

Dear Doctor:
    I feel I must write for myself, and for my Age Mates. I am sorry it seems necessary. Actually, I wonder what will

happen to me should I fall into the hands of someone who reads this and wants revenge. However, I feel a greater responsibility on behalf of my "fellow" women. Once we get sick, you have all the power, and it frightens us.

I would never have known that doctors discriminate had I not been a member of the Medical Faculty Wives Club for three and a half decades. As the wife of an influential doctor, I knew hundreds of you. Entertained you in my home, mixed buckets of cocktails, prepared midnight lunches and often listened to your young troubles. Throughout all those years you gave me thoughtful, considerate medical care, always with the approval of my husband.

Today my situation is significantly different. I fear having to consult you professionally. Since I am now just an aging female, and no longer connected to the circle of colleagues, you treat me poorly. You dismiss my questions with platitudes. You look down on me. You avoid having to touch my body even diagnostically, preferring blood samples, X-rays and biopsies.

You tend to assume I am a hypochondriac. You sometimes write judgmental, even snide referral letters to your colleagues. You keep me waiting for hours, assuming my time is without value. You drug me unnecessarily and often without regard to previously prescribed medication. You do not adequately explain the side effects of drugs, and don't listen when I tell you I have had previous experience with some of the worst of them.

I can't escape the feeling that you don't like me. I am the same person I was a few years ago, just older. I ask you to think about your attitude toward age in general, and especially aging women. Your honored oath admonishes you to treat all patients with equal respect. My charge is that you do not always do so. When you are unable to take my concerns seriously, couldn't you refer me to someone I can talk to, someone who provides less medicalized treatment? I need information on body changes now that I am growing older. Maybe massage to ease aching joints and muscles. I need to know how to handle stress, exercise, diet and bereavement. I know you don't have time to treat sick lives, but you could help me find those who can. I require something more than a routine tranquilizer.

Most of my Age Mates concur in these feelings but are afraid to speak out. We tend to see the treatment we receive as discrimination, as sexism. Although ageism may be based on compassion not ill will, a patronizing attitude is destructive to a person's self-confidence.

We want to trust you, feel safe in your care. Perhaps you should remember that one of our numbers took care of you when you were incontinent, drooling, helpless, and that we contributed to the society that provided you with medical training facilities, and opportunity. However hard you studied or however much you paid as tuition, it was only a drop in the bucket of the real costs the whole society contributed to make you into a doctor. As a last thought, maybe we should remind you that you are going to be old too, and you should start now to do unto others as you would be done by.

You are the only one who can change yourself. Think back to the high ideals which motivated you to study for the profession, and as healer/physician help us better utilize our capacity to heal ourselves.

CHOOSING A DOCTOR

It is best to choose a physician when you are healthy. The better a doctor knows your background and medical history, the easier it will be to provide effective treatment when you need it. Start by asking friends, neighbors, and especially Age Mates, whom they see and if they are satisfied with their care, as well as the doctor's treatment and philosophy. If you are new to a community, call the College of Physicians and Surgeons and ask them to provide the names of three physicians in the area who are accepting new patients.

The second step is to make an appointment to *interview* the physician. It's a good idea to write down the questions you want to ask. Talk to the doctor, try to sense his or her approach to medical treatment. Is it focused on wellness, on prevention, and health maintenance? Where does the doctor have hospital privileges? Does she or he undertake surgery in preference to more conservative treatment? Is there a willingness to discuss your concerns? What does your intuition tell you? Do you trust him or her? Are you comfortable talking with that particular doctor?

In selecting a doctor, find out above all if she or he will be your advocate. Will the doctor represent *your* best interests in times of crises, in case of accident, medical complications, referral to surgery, admission to long-term care facility? Will he or she consider your rights in cases of interference from family? These are some of the more general considerations. Your particular medical needs may require other qualifications. Don't be afraid to ask! Finally, if you are not confident with your doctor's assessment or treatment of your condition, get another opinion.

Given the similarity of medical instruction, and the tight regulations enforced by the American and Canadian Medical Associations, you can be more or less sure that any doctor in practice has been well trained in conventional medicine. She or he will vary in experience, but basic training will be essentially the same. Look at the diplomas, by all means. And do see if there is a woman doctor to interview. I suggest you also interview one or more doctors not trained in North America. They will have been required to fulfill an internship acquainting them with Western medical practices, machines, and so on, but there is often something in their attitude toward patients that is comforting.

Doctors in other cultures seem to honor the patient as well as treat the presenting disease. I base this on having worked with a number of postdoctoral fellows from outside North America, and on the Pakistani doctor who tended my father through his long terminal illness. He never failed to *care* even when he knew he could no longer help. He informed and comforted my mother throughout the six-month ordeal, and explained to all of us as much as he knew. For the rest of her life he continued to look in on her whenever he came through my home town.

In making your choice, the basis of your decision will not be the prestige of the medical degree, the nationality or gender, but whether you feel you can trust your physician. Your care will be even more satisfactory if you also like the doctor.

REAL HEALTH

Statisticians, and particularly politicians, tend to measure "health" by the availability of doctors and medical facilities within a given jurisdiction. Supposedly one garners zillions of votes by building new hospitals. But health is far more than hospitalization or the number of visits we make to the doctor. Physicians render invaluable service when they are able to "fix" an ailment, but the actual cure originates from the inner strength of the living person. With all their pills and potions and surgical procedures, the medical profession can only assist the body to heal itself.

In Sweden, where a larger percentage of citizens reach sixty-five than in any other country, they speak of *thrivsil*, a word with no accurate English translation. It means a combination of the desire to live and the joy of thriving. Where there is a will, life thrives despite seemingly impossible handicaps. We are inspired by stories of people who refuse to be victimized by life-threatening ailments. These people, many of them Age Mates, find the inner strength to triumph over the loss of limbs, sight, mobility or hearing, to create a life well worth living. Others run to a doctor acting as if they might perish from terminal hangnail.

We must evaluate the cost-effectiveness of a wide range of health and medical measures, and make decisions on how best to use existing facilities in the interest of healthier, more fulfilling lives. To accomplish this rewarding objective, sentient patients must assume responsibility for their own well-being, and be aware of their rights, including the right to die with dignity. The doctor, overworked, specialized, possibly distracted by more interesting patients, must examine his attitudes, and recognize that there may be beneficial non-medical treatments. Perhaps he will need to relinquish some of his closely guarded territory and let in others more able to help those whose problems are based in disappointment, sorrow, loneliness and a disrupted life. For this challenging task the medical system will need to recruit some apprentice gods. Much in medical care depends on the doctor's humanity, for, as in the time of the ancients, medicine remains as much an art as a science.

CHAPTER 10

GOOD MEDICINE

L iving beings have within their bodies a pharmacopoeia of good medicine. Our internal treatment centre can lower blood pressure, calm heart rate, soothe nerves, regulate digestion, manage elimination, heal wounds and keep us functioning through life's thick and thin—all qualities to help preserve us into great old age. Considerable research is being devoted to understanding the body's self-healing resources—"discoveries" of what we have long known in our hearts.

The time is at hand to consciously apply the body's healing capacity to our own lives. Knowing that the good medicine is accessible is the first step, knowing where to find it is the second, and calling it into use is the third. We have known about good medicine all along. It's that extra ounce of strength, that chancy insight, that ability to ease someone's else's pain and sorrow. This good medicine is generated from common sense, life experience and love. It is what mothers do.

> When it comes to the health of the people, I would rather a troupe of clowns entered the city than a caravan loaded with all the drugs of Egypt.   —Old Eastern Proverb

Norman Cousins, a well-known writer, documented his conscientious pursuit of laughter to conquer a life-threatening brain tumor. Told he had only months to live, and with much work still undone, he decided he would, at least, die laughing. He rented all the funny movies he had ever heard of, movies there hadn't been time to see in his busy, productive life. So he watched, laughed at the craziness and in time, actually laughed the tumor into remission. Impossible? The doctors thought so, but could hardly doubt the evidence. With Cousins' remarkable results and his ongoing inspiration, researchers set out to discover how laughter cured.

Apparently joyful, rollicking, tear-shedding laughter stimulates the body to produce the mysterious healing substances, *endorphins*, which stimulate activity of the immune system.

Patients at a San Francisco convalescent home were able to substantially reduce their doses of painkillers after four weeks of playing a game in which they took turns making each other laugh. Family jokes, though cursed by strangers, are a bond which keeps families together. If it's good for a laugh, and not at someone's expense, it's good medicine.

A hearty laugh—the kind that makes your eyes tear and your stomach hurt—can de-stress you just as well as relaxation and better than tranquilizers, according to Sabina White of the Laughter Project at the University of California, Santa Barbara. Her workshops focus on sharing embarrassing moments and laughing about them, learning ways to find humor in distressing situations, and talking about the kinds of humor that are healing—such as jokes about life. She also studied the kinds that *aren't* healing: hurtful jokes that put down groups of people. Crude "jokes" about women and minorities apparently increase stress rather than ameliorate it—in both men and women! Humor, like other forms of communication, benefits from political correctness.

Seek out funny stuff. Librarians and booksellers will have suggestions. Look at cartoons and comics—some of them *are* amusing. Rent comedy videos, read books and poems by humorists, and for the sheer nonsense of it, find a copy of *MAD* magazine. Grab yourself a look-back-in-laughter experience. Alfred E. Newman is as goofy as when our kids sneaked him home, and the jokes are just as silly. *MAD* is more than thirty years old!!

An experience of laughter, especially before bedtime, helps assure sound sleep. In any event it is wiser to spend casual time laughing than immersed in the sorrows of fictional characters. You might catch their diseases! I've watched some television shows laughing like a child in a Hall of Mirrors. They can be hilarious!

Why do we laugh at certain things—pratfalls, trip-ups, mistaken identities, people falling into water, or the discomfiture of men whose pants fall down? Maybe our laughter reflects our inordinate pride in being two-legged animals. That's pretty funny in itself. Perhaps vaudeville isn't dead at all; it just moved to television.

Laughter is the most fun when it is shared. An audience is stimulated to ongoing hilarity when it is tuned in to a "running gag" and everyone laughs together. Then there are the clowns who have been with us since the beginning—the jesters, comedians, mimes, buffoons—who bind kings and commoners together. These creatures of laughter are the other side of life's two-way mirror. Clowns brought laughter to the Roman Forum and to the present rodeo. Beware of those who would denounce clowns.

Some Age Mates tell me they almost never laugh. Unless they get a refresher course in joy, they are in immediate danger of getting old. Good-humored people infect others with joyful spirits, and are much more interesting to be around. Quite incidentally they also lower stress in themselves and others. In a world so beset with conflict and power trips it may take some effort to reawaken the lighter side of life, but it is worth a try. Even some bottom-line corporations are creating opportunities for employees to have fun. They find that productivity increases, absenteeism decreases and people enjoy their jobs more. So it is with life. All work and no play *does* make us dull.

We need mirth. Shared jokes, amusing sayings and gag lines are all part of the "really big shew" that unifies a people. Few cultures survive in good health without sharing joy and laughter, and many have survived incredible obstacles because of their ability to find humor in adversity. The heritage of humor, along with songs, stories, dances and celebrations, are the epoxy of communities. A gift of laughter is valuable to giver and givee. For my own good, I keep telling myself to lighten up. Taking life too seriously may be hazardous to your health. Some say the reason angels fly is because they take themselves so lightly.

> Time flies when you're having fun. Or, as the frog said to
> her companion, "Time is fun when you're having flies."

"Cats are people too, you know!" Or so a four-year-old told me. Most of us know from childhood that it is nice to have pets. A pet to greet one's homecoming is life-affirming. Something reassuring happens when we stroke a warm, soft living creature. A few minutes spent petting an animal actually lowers an elevated blood pressure. We become calm, breathe more deeply, relax, smile, and with any luck, laugh. A pet is an excellent counselor, always respecting confidentiality. When resentment fills the air, a friendly nudge by cat or dog deflects the tension. We sometimes shed tears into the soft fur. Taking responsibility for a living creature gives shape to our days. Pets encourage exercise and return our attention with loyal companionship and amusement.

It may reassure you to learn that pets and people are now a subject for study. Pets are companions, partners, friends who accept us as we are without judgment. They expect little beyond devoted attention and the care we give them as their right.

It has probably been this way since God was a woman, for it is thought we domesticated the species that lived near us by feeding and caring for young animals who had been abandoned, or whose mothers were killed in the hunt. Through the ages, people and animals have enjoyed a kind of symbiosis, an interspecies relationship that connects us, however tenuously, to the non-human world. It is believed our ancestors relied on animals to signal impending dangers such as earthquakes. Until quite recently canaries were carried down into the mines to warn of dangerous gases. And, just as a precaution, I don't eat mushrooms from the forest until I know some living creature has taken a bite out of the same species. It seems certain that the disappearing species of our days are also warning us of danger.

Animals are specially welcome in places where humans are confined. Cats and dogs are going to prisons and rest homes in thousands of facilities across North America, to the joy of the people who live there.

Studies have concluded that pets are an incentive to get well faster and even to live longer. The loyalty and affection of a familiar animal allows us to weep tears of sorrow or thanksgiving. The creatures manifest empathy, knowing who is a friend and who needs a friend. The healing power of animals stimulates spirit and body and connects us with the Earth. A person at home recovering from a heart attack has a statistically better chance of surviving more than one year if there's an animal complicating his or her life.

But you can't just order up an affectionate pussycat with french fries to go. Like any other kind of friend, her personality must be respected. Don't expect to enjoy a frisky puppy if you have trouble keeping up, or a huge dog if you are afraid of falling, and think twice about either if you are houseproud. There are fashions in animals as in operations. Avoid choosing a pet for insincere reasons. A creature you truly like will share your life and soon know more about you than you know yourself.

People have dogs; cats have people. Dogs require a master and return obedient allegiance and undying affection. Cats tend to lead independent lives. Our senior animal, Pizzicato (Pitzi for short), has appeared with me in publicity photos and has received her own fan mail. We now have a second animal—sent, I believe, to complicate and improve my life. She arrived entirely by accident. A friend insisted I go for a walk on our rocky beach, even though it was one of my arthritic days and I was using my cane. We had gone only a few feet when we heard a small, wild cry. There amid the driftwood was a tiny, scrawny orange creature. She was scrambling over the huge obstacles, trying to reach someone. Her fur was stiff with seawater and she was frantically thirsty. Apparently someone had tried to drown her. For her heroic five week-old survival efforts we named her Magnificat, "Maggie" for short. Incidentally, I forgot my cane on the beach. Maggie greatly enriches our lives, so much so that we assure visitors we are not just a couple of seniors dotty over a cat, but that we are studying inter-species communication. Sure, that too.

The cats apparently own our house. They go in and out their door at will, and never permit anything, especially squirrels or the neighbor's cat, to come near it. Pitzi continues to stroll her tiny path through the patchy grass to the beach where she sits and meditates, staring out to sea. On rainy days this practical animal watches the passing parade with her head out the cat door, her behind comfortably settled in the warmth of the house. Maggie is not allowed to do this, since Pitzi guards her privileges. Except for a short period of confusion when Daylight Savings Time comes or goes, it is possible to tell the hour by their arrival for dinner. When we humans find ourselves in conflict, we can often bridge the communication gap by talking to, or caring for, these remarkably independent creatures who adopted us, their little cat suitcases packed with as much love and laughter as we can hold. Sharing the affection and dependence of an animal is a tie that binds. They don't, however, know who is likely to sneeze in honor of their presence.

When it is impossible to keep a furry pet, think fish. Watching the lazy, graceful movements of fish is a soothing way to pass the time. The aquarium in a dentist's or doctor's office has more than a decorative function. The compulsory twenty to thirty minutes of waiting spent gazing at an aquarium can relax people as effectively as hypnosis!

If you don't want to tend an aquarium, try bird watching! It is the most popular sport in North America, with millions of participants. Phone around to find a flock of "birders" and join in. I know one Age Mate in a wheel chair who is never without her binoculars, whether she is out in the park or at home near a window. Good exercise, fresh air, interesting focus of attention, and good medicine!

Speaking of fresh air—the joys and benefits of gardening are many. Green, living "creatures" brighten the home, and it has recently been discovered that some species—easy-to-grow spider plants, for example—have the ability to cleanse the air of rotten things like smoke and odors, restoring health-giving oxygen to reward our care. The greening of offices and homes is a fairly recent trend and workers miss plants when they are not there.

My first house plant experience took place in a dismal basement flat when, by chance, I put a sprouting sweet potato in a jar of water on one of the two narrow window sills. It rewarded me with a lush cascade of green as long as I lived there. Plants are great for giving to friends, trading, and starting conversations. (And incidentally, you *can* talk to your plants. Several research types have confirmed that plants benefit. None of them mentioned that humans benefit too.) Studying a seed catalog in the depths of winter is great recreation even if you have little expectation of prize-winning blooms or two-pound carrots.

Plants are also of the Earth, living things that respond to intelligent care, adaptable to almost any human condition. Gardens, should you be one of the lucky people with land at their disposal, provide challenge and satisfaction, as well as fruits and flowers. Among a garden's most important rewards are color, pure food and exercise in the fresh air. Some communities have garden plots for rent where vegetables, flowers and friendships bloom.

Many of these are specially geared to people with impaired mobility.

The garden associated with the home was developed in medieval times so sequestered women could have a place to roam. The great formal, walled gardens of courts, convents and palaces were often the only opportunity for women to be outside "taking the air." Our freedom to dig, plant, cultivate and harvest for our own pleasure is worth honoring.

Composting waste vegetation is an authentic miracle. How grass clippings, weeds, leaves and peelings turn themselves into lovely, rich brown soil never ceases to amaze me. Learn about organic gardening, and how other living creatures—insects, earthworms, toads, snakes, butterflies—serve the garden, and the fertility of Earth. All life is made of the same stuff.

The worst thing about being 65 is that I don't have any fun.

Quite a few Age Mates have told me that. It's not that we can't have fun after sixty, but that we've forgotten to take fun seriously. Duty and the Calvinist work ethic erected monstrous walls to keep us from appreciating play—and keep us from liveliness too, for that matter!

Play, in its anthropological sense, is the place to try out different roles, ideas, things, personae, clothes and so on, to see how it feels or just for the fun of it. Remember dressing up as nurses, teachers and lovely ladies, acting out the parts, using the props, inventing the speech we thought our make-believe selves would use? We tried this out at the Amazing Grays gathering. We dressed up in whatever special clothes we had with us and made crowns of ivy, flowers, and sometimes sparkling things to honor our Cronehood. Almost all of us entered the game and except for a very few who thought the rest of us were silly, we had a wonderful moment of make-believe. Some of the women rediscovered the child within.

Adults should remember that play permits human beings to

experiment. The ideas for countless discoveries have come from "just fooling around." We dig ruts for ourselves by doing things over and over in the same old way. Our institutions do the same, repeating old un-thinking routines, when imagination could create more satisfying ways of being. We can miss life that way.

North American culture, in its fixation on the bottom line, seeks the *end*, rarely considering the *way* as anything more than an impediment. Going from point to point in any undertaking eliminates the *how* of getting where you want to go, and missing many of the discoveries and pleasures. Playing with ideas generated from thinking up and throwing out, doing and discarding, evaluating and deciding, keeps the inquiring mind in trim. We need not always have a set purpose or foresee a finished end-product. We can just play with stuff to see what happens, and for the sheer joy of messing about.

Play has a bad image in a culture which says we should be out making money. In some places we don't dare enjoy our jobs or the boss will think we don't work hard enough. The production line mentality discourages imagination and individuality. Sadly we have mostly relegated play to children, musical instruments, or commercial enterprises like football and slot machines.

Actually, play is the cradle of creativity. It is where we dare to dream and explore for ourselves, and for our inner child. Play may reveal the kernel of new ways of doing. Without it we get bogged down in lifeless ruts of habit. Creativity is energizing. Where the creative process flows without prejudgment, it twists and frolics to reveal new spaces, new ways of seeing, with no particular time frame, no set end result, and no right or wrong way. Play enhances life.

At the summer solstice a group of women in my community hold a potluck feast with flowers and candles to celebrate the longest day of the year. The custom honoring Midsummer Day goes back to the beginning of human time so we dress up as goddesses! Since goddesses are everywhere, immanent, in every possible form, we are free to devise whatever personality or costume we might imagine. We learn about the qualities of our goddess so that we can tell the group, and invent appropriate headdresses of vines, flowers and symbols to portray her.

The first year I was far too shy to make-believe about anything, and that was all right too. But last year I wrapped myself in an emerald-green sari, wove a wreath of leaves and flowers, carried blades of new grain, and spoke as Mother Earth, the goddess, Gaia. Taking on so powerful a persona was uplifting, empowering.

Art is the cure for chaos—taking assortments of unrelated, chaotic thoughts, sounds, materials and organizing them into order. Get out some pencils, paints or crayons and just "goof around." Scissors, old magazines, bits of cloth, glue and tape supply hours of exploration trying shapes, colors and textures this way and that. Play with the materials for the fun of it, alone or with friends. Make a collage about your life. And don't worry about masterpieces. It is the nature of creativity that one always does the best one can do. As for making the "best" collage, forget it. You absolutely *have* to make the first effort before you can attempt a second, which you may like better. There is no right or wrong way to make art—just your way. Perfection has no place in art's intention; it just happens. Art is in the hands of the Muses.

Try drawing or painting again. Let your shapes be bold with the experience of your years. Color outside the lines! Or reconsider the fiber arts that interest you. Think knitting, sewing, embroidery, tatting, crocheting, weaving, hooking, needlepoint, cutwork, quilting, appliqué and on and on. All can be channels for creative expression. The doing keeps you supple and can even delay arthritic fingers.

To gain a whole new appreciation of the value and variety of women's arts, ask your library to get any of Judy Chicago's books on how her work, *The Dinner Party*, was made. *The Dinner Party* is a life-size sculpture of a table with settings for women who, throughout history, have contributed to women's culture. It is one of the outstanding artistic accomplishments of our time, and it is all about women and centuries of their accomplishments. Women's talents have clothed us, brought beauty into our homes, enriched our lives and kept us warm in winter. Don't worry about the way some people denigrate women's arts. A certain husband I once knew said he approved of women knitting—"It gives them something to think about while talking." I'll bet he wears store-bought socks now.

When you are engaged in creative activities, your body responds in remarkable ways. Blood pressure goes down, your mind opens up, details become visible, and you feel better. In addition to the physiological changes of the moment, you will probably live longer! Think how many composers, painters, poets, conductors and musicians live to a ripe old age, continuing to enrich their lives and ours with their creativity. No one needs an excuse to engage in such wellness-promoting activities, just do it. You have about twenty-five years to finish the project!

Have you thought about toys to play with? You're entitled! We hear about men who finally get the model train of their dreams. Women have similar dreams. One friend, a very busy television writer, had always wanted a dollhouse. Her grown-up kids built one for her fiftieth birthday. She delights herself making little drapes, upholstering miniature furniture, weaving tiny rugs. Friends gave her a dollhouse-warming and brought little gifts. She is often away on business trips and chases spare-time loneliness by searching for just the right tiny things to furnish the dollhouse. It is her hobby and her grandchildren love it.

Hobbies provide a focus for ongoing interests, and can be anything or everything that isn't "work" work. Some women do fancy cooking, make bread, weave tapestries, grow lovely flowers, raise guppies, search antique stores, all as hobbies. Others collect stamps, stories, plates, coins or spoons. A hobby can be anything from learning languages to helping out at art galleries or hospitals. Any activity that turns *you* on becomes endlessly fascinating as you grow in understanding and adventurousness. We also become "interesting" in direct proportion to the interest we show in other people and other ideas. Interesting people have more fun.

I called on an Age Mate to exchange some pottery supplies. After inviting me in she made me promise I wouldn't laugh if she introduced me to her friend. "I want you to meet my companion, Herbert." I didn't know what or whom to expect. She said, "He's always sitting there with an impish grin, waiting until I come home, and the management doesn't object. I always say hello in case he has decided to listen. When danceable music comes on the radio I grab Herbert and dance him around. He never steps on my toes, doesn't complain about the hours I keep or harp on my short-comings. Sometimes on cold nights I even take him to bed with me. It's nice to have something warm to cuddle. He doesn't snore or care if I kick him out."

She had bought herself a real toy, a large, soft teddy bear! We deserve to treat ourselves once in a while. Someday I may be flush enough to get a real porcelain doll with a gorgeous dress and soft, curly hair. At least it is fun looking.

Out in the wider community there are thousands of important tasks that can only be done by volunteers with experience in living. Alfred N. Larsen, national director of the federal US Retired Senior Volunteer Program (RSVP), has placed hundreds of thousands of elderly people in community volunteer jobs. (Keep in mind that "elderly" is anyone over fifty-five!) He is convinced of the value of volunteer work as people grow older. For those who lose family or friends, assisting others helps restore purpose to living. Generosity has valuable paybacks. We reap the love and gratitude we inspire in those we help. Like stress, love has a cumulative effect.

When you volunteer, seek to harmonize your interests with the interests of the community. Put your energy into tasks *you* enjoy, not where you think you *should*. Every outreach organization needs help. If your interest is in the arts, volunteer at a local gallery, get to meet the artists, act as hostess for openings, help hang exhibitions. If you miss being around children, check out mentoring or story telling in the schools, cuddling the newborns at hospitals or being a Big Sister to some young girl. In any event, do *your* thing because that is what you will do best, and what you can do most meaningfully for others.

People who engage in volunteer work enjoy better health, visit the doctor less often and have fewer physical and emotional complaints. Service to others keeps us youthful. Caring for others actually keeps us alive. Women know this instinctively. It is our life work, and could be one of the reasons for our longer life expectancy.

It has been suggested that altruism through the ages has contributed to the survival of the human species. Throughout our time on Earth, people have lived in tribes and small groups. Natural selection demanded that we evolve as creatures willing to help, rescue and protect others of our group. We developed empathy for others. Age Mates are experienced in solving conflicts, a skill greatly needed in today's world. Much good is done when we put ourselves in another's shoes and care for others as we would be cared for. Think of the millions of people helped through UNICEF, other millions through various volunteer campaigns—United Way, Salvation Army, the Peace Corps, Red Cross, Canada's CUSO, and that special women's overseas support group, MATCH.

> I was looking for a pet charity, and I found MATCH. It gives tiny loans to help third world women set up small businesses, purchase seeds, etc. For about the cost of a Big Mac, a woman in Africa or Asia can buy enough garden seeds to supplement her family's diet. The program is very successful, and it gives me a good woman-to-woman feeling.

I often think, "There but for the grace of God go I." The
bank takes ten dollars out of my account every month. It
really isn't missed from my pension. Every so often the
MATCH Bulletin reports on remarkable accomplishments
by women with access to loans as small as $25 or $50. I care
about those faraway women, and send them my blessing.

—Age Mate, 67

Meaningful charity involves more than money and more than
Brownie points awarded for good deeds. The *giver* reaps the
benefits of giving when the urge comes from the goodness in her
heart. I know one Age Mate who feels a kind of "high" from helping
out in a nursing home, and others who say that doing something
nice for someone snapped them out of periods of depression.
Volunteering can make you feel better about yourself, give you a
new sense of purpose, and even find friends.

A neighbor who loves driving, but doesn't enjoy going alone, has
found pleasure in driving two very old women to places of scenic
beauty. "I get to see places I've never seen before and hear their
stories about the old days," she says. A long-distance grandmother
filled a great yearning as a volunteer cuddler in the hospital
nursery. Another said, "I've been taking my sleepy little dog to a
nursing home every other Tuesday for most of a year. Everyone
wakes up including the dog. He loves the attention. So do I!"

Now that we realize that Earth herself urgently needs our
care, hundreds of us have found a new lease on life in our work
with environmental organizations. We get the "helper's high"
from believing that we can make a difference to the kind of
world we leave our grandchildren. At the very least, we learn to
live more lightly on the Earth and return something to this
cherished place.

Tears wash trouble away. They help heal the body and the soul.
Suppressed sorrow can become a festering sore. Let it out. If you

keep a hurt inside it remains forever imprinted somewhere deep down. The body never forgets. Sorrow, pain, grief, disappointment can hang around from childhood. When the hurt is acknowledged and honored, tears will help dissolve it. When a book or a movie touches a sensitive place in your heart, let the tears come rather than shoving your feelings away, getting all tight and plugged up. Tears release pent-up emotions in much the same way as dreams. Crying "gets it out of your system" as the old saying goes. We know how a good cry can cleanse, how it restores calm to a troubled heart.

Like laughter, tears release healing chemicals secreted through the tear glands and carried by the bloodstream to all parts of the body. For instance, tears have been shown to have a positive effect on skin repair. This may be one reason why children, still willing to shed their tears, heal so much more rapidly than tearless adults.

The traditional stiff upper lip, esteemed by many, was invented by the military to enable superior officers to chew out inferior ranks without fear of reprisals, and to cloak cadets' emotions. Transferring a stiff upper lip to normal daily activities closes down on life. It may help you conform to someone else's expectations, but it will leave you with knots inside. Let the healing tears flow. Let them ease hurt and sorrow away. And may your tears also celebrate hours of joy, rejoicing in a heart full to overflowing. Humans weep.

"Music hath charms to soothe the savage breast," said William Congreve in 1695, and despite the raucous sound barrage of some contemporary "music," he is still right. Music is good medicine. Dr. Blair Justice, author of *Who Gets Sick*, advises:

> When you feel as if you're coming down with something, listen to music that really moves you. It can't guarantee that you won't get sick, since illness isn't caused just by the mind. But the mind can help resist illness, and exposing

yourself to beauty is one of the best ways to develop resisters.

—from Bricklin et al, *Positive Living and Health*

One of the finest things human beings can do on this Earth is to make harmonious sounds together. Music bonds us. A group of people together in music responds to the same rhythm, feels the rise and fall of the same melody. Anthropological and historical evidence reveals that devices for making music have been around for at least thirty thousand years. No matter how complex or simple, every culture makes music. It is said to be a gift of the gods.

The nine Muses, descended from the primordial Triple Goddess, are still with us, safeguarding the wonder of human creation. Revered by the ancient Greeks, the Muses were the source of "in-spiration," literally breathing in the "music of the spheres." Without any of our sophisticated measuring instruments, the ancients knew that sound radiates outward on waves that become spheres, encompassing all that is. Music is the symbolic expression of the vibrations within each living being.

We often experience the way music is used to stir loyalties during patriotic moments, how it reinforces and builds to enhance action on the screen. People sing their faith, proclaim hope or victory, lament sorrow, or soothe a child to sleep. Music is a distinctly human quality.

The most ancient of all musical instruments is the human voice. Joined with others, these ancestral talents elaborate into choral music involving people all over the world, blending hearts and voices to create transcendent sound. Remember the family "choir" gathered around piano, organ, ukulele, violin, accordion or harmonica in Grandma's parlor? These were major sources of music before technology came up with Victrolas, crystal sets, stereos, wrap-around sound and digital recordings. In the old way it didn't matter very much whether or not you were off-key.

Being part of a choir is good medicine, and it also makes good community. Confidence soars with music and time shines brighter. Find a choir to join, or start one yourself. You may want to set up a group of irrepressible Raging Grannies to give voice to your satirical, political or environmental concerns, as well as share the gift of laughter and good fun with onlookers.

Nearly everyone wishes they could play a musical instrument or regrets having given one up. Why not start again, or for the first time? I know a group of men over seventy calling themselves Gray Jazz. They play the great tunes of our youth—Glen Miller, Cole Porter, the Dorseys and others. They are fantastic! Memories surge to the surface, and we can hear them on cassette.

Playing an instrument stimulates both the creative and logical parts of the brain and requires them to interact. It exercises co-ordination between eye and hand. Playing an instrument helps you retain mental lucidity in later years, and dispenses lifelong joy. And just wait until you can play or sing with grandchildren!

Those ancient Muses wander even through the turmoil of our times. Search for them to comfort your soul. All of art is good medicine. Give words to your own thoughts and dreams—write your own stories and poems. Take in a play. A concert. A recital. Go to or give a literary reading. Visit an art gallery to see beautiful sculpture and paintings, or try to figure out why the ugly ones are there. If you know what you like, search your mind to find out why you like it, and then explore other possibilities.

Appropriate music is an asset to meditation, healing, exercise, digestion and lovemaking. Sing with the vacuum cleaner, while walking, washing dishes, weeding the garden and in the bath. Make your own kind of music, sing your own kind of song, no matter who else sings along.

All life dances! It begins with the circular dance inside the atom, reaches into human activity from every culture, transforms great social movements, and eventually manifests itself in the super-vigorous rock concerts fancied by our children and grandchildren. The kinesthetic experience of dance releases the body and gives physical expression to emotions. Dance acts out the hunt, celebrates the harvest, glorifies birth, consecrates human events, solemnizes death. We see this in the ceremonies of North American native people, and we watched the epic changes in South Africa as people danced their grief and their triumph. We lose something of importance when the language of dance fades from our lives. Dance is something we do *now*. It is a complete exercise uniting body, mind and spirit. Even the most conservative will recall how King David danced. Movement transformed into dance unites, celebrates and renews.

Somehow our culture has lost dance as an ingredient in celebrations. The ceremonial dance once fixed the sacredness of life into the body memory, uniting young and old, women and men in shared rhythm, affirming the group's cohesiveness. In our dominant culture's determination not to have any fun, too many of us turned dancing into a formal affair with invitations, set routines and romantic overtones. About all the dancing most of us do as adults are fleeting remnants at New Year's Eve and maybe weddings. There *are* square dances, barn dances, street dances, line dances, and sometimes dancing on the green, which is the most fun of all. We should look until we find the dancers and join in. Or invite our own!

There are few if any set dance forms these days, no complex steps to learn, and no "right" way of doing any of the movements. Many of us would not venture out on the dance floor in our youth unless we had a suitable partner or knew the precise steps devised by Arthur Murray. We aren't obliged to have partners now. It is acceptable, possibly becoming traditional, to dance alone, absorbing the rhythm, marking the beat, with the music of the spheres seeping in.

My personal favorite, barring the unlikely possibility of going to a real dance, is to get up and "cut a rug" while the commercials play on television. In the beginning my joints were more grunt-and-groan than rock-and-roll but things are getting looser!

Dancing to commercials is an energizing interlude for the so-called couch potato. We can take sweet revenge on those intrusions into modern life. A vigorous or graceful interval of full body movement while commercials provide the rhythm is a useful antidote to the stress we accumulate during long periods of sitting. If your mobility is impaired, remember that you can "dance" with every moving part of you!

Make opportunities to dance. Ritual dance is open to everyone, each dancer doing what comes naturally through the music. The necessity to dance in couples went out with the Twist. But it is such a pity so many men get old before *our* time. A woman fortunate enough to know a good male dance partner is thrice blest. Something totally wonderful happens when dancers move together in each others' arms.

Some churches bring worship and dancing together. A few years ago I attended a gospel service at an African Methodist Church in Vancouver. Along with two hundred or more men, women, young, old, black, white and in-between, I was up on my feet dancing with the congregation, feeling the exultation of the music. It was glorious. There we were, the happy crowd of us, crammed together in pews. We all felt refreshed as we reluctantly headed home.

Make occasions to enjoy the grace of dancers, figure skaters, athletes. The body unconsciously imitates their movements. Notice how your body responds even if you are unable to be part of the dance. The beat of the drum is irresistible to all but the most inert. You can scarcely avoid walking in time with a marching band or responding to the heartbeat rhythms of Native drummers.

Dance to your own drummer. Make up the steps. Let any or all parts of your body respond, not caring what others think. Dance with each other as you did when you were young. Dance holding a grandchild, a teddy bear, your cane, a bouquet of flowers, or with your own special self. Feel how your body responds, notice the change in your heartbeat, your breathing and, above all, your happiness. We reconnect with the circle dance of atoms, for life itself is the Dance!

Chapter 11

Walk to the Fountain of Youth

The trouble with doing nothing is you never get a day off.
—Old saying

With exercise we flower and become. Without it we wither and die. Exercise may be our *best* medicine. The human body was created to move, to do, to act, and when we stop doing, the bones, joints, and circulation more or less seize up. It may even be that women live longer than men because of our ongoing activity. We are always getting up to get something, bending over to pick things up, getting things out of drawers and reaching up or down in kitchen cupboards. We pull weeds or pick flowers, and reach up to clean, dust, whatever. Older men don't do much of that sort of thing, and so apparently they go to seed faster. What a fabulous opportunity for us to get help with the housework!

Regular physical activity is important at all ages. It allows growing children to develop strong muscles, bones and flexible joints. Exercise increases the efficiency and endurance of the heart, lungs and muscles. Movement helps maintain these same

178

essentials in mature people, helps with posture, balance and co-ordination, and maintains the strength of bones. It helps us handle stress, reduces fatigue, promotes better sleep, and provides the person who exercises with a sense of well-being and zest for life. A very recent study informs us that regular exercise, particularly in younger women, helps prevent breast cancer.

Few experiences compare with the sensuous pleasure of a good stretch. Feel your body in all its extremities. Stretch everything you can whenever you think about it, but always in the morning. Start the day with the pleasures of long stretches, deep breaths and healthy wake-up yawns to stretch the face. It keeps muscles in condition and prevents injury and soreness. A large percentage of accidents occur in the early morning, and although I have never seen a reason for this finding, joints and muscles stiffen during a night's inactivity, and it seems likely that they fail to respond as we expect them to when we are fully awake.

Wake up slowly and do a good set of isometric exercises under the covers in the warmth of your bed. Make up a routine which involves all the big muscles you can safely move, and which gently twists your back. Lace your fingers together behind your neck, point elbows to the ceiling, then gently turn the torso first to the left and then the right. Press your back to the bed, hold and repeat. Stretch one leg after the other as far toward the end of the bed as possible to loosen up the pelvis. Pull your knees up to your chest if it doesn't cause a domestic disturbance, or invite your partner to join the routine. But do it your way. Get out of bed carefully and check your balance. One of the perks of maturity is that we usually don't have to jump out of bed to catch a bus or impress anyone, so take your time. It is one of the privileges of age! So are afternoon naps, incidentally.

Age Mates have been quick to recognize the advantages of regular exercise. More seniors are enrolled in exercise classes than any other age group. We know the human body must move. Energy is stored in us, and we either kill it off or let it out in constructive, health-giving ways. In recent years, renewed interest in the importance of exercise at all ages has resulted in a variety of options—aerobics, bodybuilding, lifting weights, gym and swim classes, jogging, yoga and Tai Chi, to mention only a few. Many of them can easily be adapted as our mobility lessens. Borrow a "work-out" videotape from the library (watch out for the over-strenuous ones!). If you wish to be fashion-conscious while you exercise, deck yourself out in all sorts of cute clothes in wild and wonderful colors, but that isn't necessary. The point is to be comfortably dressed to permit your body its maximum flexibility.

A good exercise program is active, not passive. Choose exercises you enjoy. For most of us it's likely to be slow and easy, although one friend of eighty-five takes off on six-day hikes in forbidding mountains and goes whitewater rafting with her nephew. Two years ago she hiked the Great Wall of China! She probably jogs. Many women report pleasure and exhilaration from jogging, but others find there are too many unchoreographed parts. Personally, I don't run anywhere unless it's necessary to get someplace in a hurry. Walking at a comfortable pace gets me there soon enough.

Walking has been called the sport of geniuses. There is something about the act of walking that does as much for your mind as for your body. Research suggests that walking strokes our brains, resulting in "increased cerebral metabolic activity." A group of sedentary people, aged fifty-five to seventy, walked on a treadmill three times a week for an hour at a time. Their physiological changes were compared with similar groups who either worked out for strength and flexibility, or who did no exercise at all. The before and after measurements revealed that aerobically trained walkers enjoyed much greater improvements in response time, visual organization, memory and mental flexibility than the others. How's that for a reason to leave the polluting car at home when you need to go to the corner store?

Since blood circulation increases, more oxygen gets to the brains of walkers. They enjoy a greater sense of vigor. There may be a shopping mall in your area which sponsors before-hours walking clubs, rain or shine. A seventy-year-old man had his picture in the paper because he had logged five thousand miles walking around a shopping mall! Another was walking twelve hundred miles to visit his daughter in the next province. Check out your community. There will be Age Mates there.

Tai Chi is one of the most complete exercises. An ancient art developed thousands of years ago in China, it is practiced daily by hundreds of thousands of people. You've probably seen it being performed on television. Nearly every program about China includes a shot of men and women going through a hand and body routine that looks much like a dance. The one hundred and eight Tai Chi movements have been honed to utter simplicity. The flowing gestures create a unity of body, mind and spirit. Over the centuries, Tai Chi movements have evolved to exercise, flex and stretch the body's muscles and joints without strain or trauma. It also improves balance.

On the theory that you can't argue with success, I thought it worth a try, and found Tai Chi both stimulating and relaxing. Indeed, it feels like a dance. All postures are done while standing which is an advantage for some of us who find the floor farther and farther away with the passing years. There are tapes, videos and classes where one can learn Tai Chi.

If you haven't tried either yoga or Tai Chi, make an occasion to do so. Both forms of movement are effective in calming the mind, enhancing body functions and relieving stress. The naturalness of the movements allows them to flow organically from one part of the body to the next, and you feel good, not sore. Your flexibility will be enhanced week by week. Both exercises can be done alone or in groups for any length of time you choose to spend. Neither drives you with a pounding rhythm, a set distance or a number to be achieved. The individual practitioner sets the pace and the tempo, relying on her body to determine the limits and the goals. Both have meditative and breathing components.

It is a personal preference, but I appreciate the sense of connectedness these ancient routines create while I'm doing them. I imagine generations, young and old, moving through the same forms in bodies like my own. It is possible they felt the same freedom and joy that movement gives, an awareness of the moment, the shared body sense of us all. Because they are natural movements, you will find yourself in a Tai Chi stretch or a yoga pose in the course of daily living. They are an extension of real life, an excellent pathway toward less stressful, more harmonious living. With all exercise, listen to your body, respect its limits and possibilities.

All movements in the vast range of activity that can be called exercise, can be found in the garden. Here you breathe fresh air, stoop, bend, stretch and reach out to touch the earth. A garden's value goes far beyond the moment, replenishing the spirit, nourishing the body and with the wisdom of conservation, returning treasure to the earth. A garden is a promise to the future, anticipation of another day when it will bear its fruits and beauty in harmony with the sun, soil, rain and your own good efforts. You can spend the winter happily dreaming your garden, building in your mind's eye the perfect visual effect, imaging lovely blossoms and plentiful zucchini. Also, it isn't necessary to weed your dreams.

Dozens of reports show that exercise is life-enhancing. Certainly it makes us feel better. Among the many alternatives, choose what *you* like to do and just do it! Experiment with several different programs. Take the sensible approach and exercise a little every day. Look for an activity you find convenient and enjoyable and begin slowly. Wear comfortable clothes and appropriate footwear. Warm up carefully and intelligently with long, full body stretches, and invigorating deep breathing. Listen to your body; pain is a signal to ease up. If you don't like a program you start with—or it doesn't like you—try something else. The important thing is to get moving. Even people with chronic diseases such as arthritis or diabetes feel better with exercise, not only in physical well-being, but emotional, mental and spiritual health as well.

Take exercise as part of good medicine whenever possible, no prescription required. You might find it handy to follow a suggestion an Age Mate in Vancouver told me about. She said she made certain to do an MBO every day. Puzzled, I asked her to explain.

> Years ago my mother told me that I was supposed to do three special things every day—something for my Mind, something for my Body and something for Others. That's an MBO!
>
> —Age Mate, 66

CHAPTER 12

GIVE US THIS DAY OUR DAILY BREAD

Give us this day our daily bread." This prayer unites all living beings. When I think of "diet," a memory from a village in India comes to mind. An elderly woman, squatting in the dust near a food distribution centre, was picking up spilled rice grains one at a time. She tucked them somehow into the palm of her hand, never dropping a single kernel. A relief worker handed her a container of clean rice which she accepted calmly with a smile and nod of thanks. She bent back to her task—picking rice grains one by one, her dignity intact.

Perhaps this is the way women gathered seeds before the dawn of agriculture. Her gaunt image has been dimmed by the frantic, often brutal scramble for bread by starving men, women and children in desperate flight across the forbidding mountains of Kurdistan, and again by the long patient lines of African refugees. I can't help but wonder which model our culture would follow in such extreme circumstances.

Taking nourishment is our most individual act. Food sustains life. The necessary act of eating is wreathed with ceremony, custom, belief and habit. What we eat is strongly determined by cultural practices which place some foods under taboo, and elevates others to ceremonial status. Some cultures maintain health with little variety and consume only a fraction of the amount we in North America eat. We all dine on elements and minerals from the Earth, yet many of us give no thought to the land that produces the food. Whatever we take into our bodies grew somewhere on the planet, the result of some evolutionary alchemy which works with sunlight to transform indigestible substances into the proteins, carbohydrates and fats which sustain life. We ingest the energy of the sun with every bite. Everything we consume is built from the raw materials of Earth and from these materials we ourselves are built.

In these times of famine or glut we are obliged to remember that eating is both a sacrament and a political act loaded with social and emotional meanings. Adele Davis's wise assertion, "You are what you eat," is more profound than was generally realized when she published her first books in the 1950s (*Let's Eat Right to Keep Fit*, *Let's Cook It Right*, etc.). She was widely scorned by the establishment, but she was ahead of her time and brought a new awareness of nutrition to many people. Her books are still worth reading for her insights and for information on how creative thinkers predict the future. Her work reminds us to take a longer look at original ideas, however unconventional.

In the bustling North American world of fast foods, cake mixes, pop tarts and pizza, everything we consider edible is immediately available in abundance, if we can pay for it. Instead of wondering where our next meal will come from, many of us worry about eating too much. North Americans seem to be obsessed with calories, convenience and cholesterol, forgetting that our food is the end product of a long series of processes which begin with living plants and animals.

I am skeptical of trendy diets published weekly. I am amused by the hyped-up pressure to get enough dietary nutrients. I am furious at an overstuffed society where millions of dollars are spent developing non-food foods so we can continue to pig out as if there were no tomorrow, or worse, no today, when half the world's people live at or near starvation. Remembering the Depression, I know we can make more intelligent arrangements.

Health and well-being depend on sensible food intake. Crucial nutritional requirements may go unnoticed in the propaganda introducing the hundreds of "new" diets. Outrageous claims create pressure to buy this or that additive-laden, non-essential chemical concoction advertised as food, its flavor masked by salt and sugar and fat.

Tasteless store-bought tomatoes hard as baseballs, perfect apples crusted with thick shiny wax, bug-free vegetables soaked in pesticides, meat hopped up with antibiotics and hormones. Rather than truth in advertising, we are subjected to propaganda telling us there is no other way and this is what we want. Wherever possible the powers that be fix us with guilt, seduce us to fit into some imagined social norm, suggest that somehow or other we will be better off if we buy their great stuff. On top of all that *North Americans pay three times as much for packaging as farmers are paid for their crops!* And the packaging ends up in overflowing landfills.

Consumers are manipulated in whatever way agribusiness and the chemical companies consider most profitable, with scant regard for negative effects on humans or the way in which our food is produced. It is estimated that the average consumer who purchases all her food from a supermarket *eats an average of six pounds of insecticides, pesticides, herbicides and hormones every year!*

It is often said "what we don't know won't hurt us," but that is not true when it comes to additives, fillers and chemicals. An Age Mate with a severe allergy to wheat must watch even the most innocent foods to avoid wheat in unexpected places. Would you believe mayonnaise? So beware. Allergies may make their first appearances as we grow older. A doctor I knew suffered fatal anaphylactic shock from drinking a glass of milk. The milk had been laced with penicillin to keep the bacteria count down.

Just when we think we understand the foods we eat, "science" rings a different bell. One day it is cholesterol—don't eat eggs, cheese, or drink whole milk because they are bad for you. Next day there are several kinds of cholesterol, and the assurance that hormone-treated beef is essential for the good life. Remember the international howl when the European Economic Community banned American beef? No one knows for sure what hormone-treated meat does, but young girls get their periods several months earlier each decade and some little boys develop breasts. Some studies suggest these changes may be the result of an excess of hormone-rich chicken and beef.

The low-cholesterol craze has been joined by a high-fiber feeding frenzy, instigated by an announcement that fiber may help reduce cholesterol *and* the possibility of colon cancer. Fiber is what we called roughage in the olden days. I will risk ridicule by suggesting that our anxiety over correct foods is a mask behind which we hide our anxiety about correct lives.

Since the end of World War Two, the food business has become highly sophisticated in manipulating its products. The list of chemicals available to processors and manufacturers grows by several thousand a year. These compounds range from a substance as benign as cornstarch to outright poisons. They exist for no purpose other than to enhance appearance, extend shelf life (which is just a way of masking staleness), or make food more appealing to the legion of dieting calorie counters. The hidden tragedy is that chemical companies, like packagers, receive a higher percentage of the food dollar than the farmers.

But there is a ray of hope for consumers who are old and smart. The general public is becoming more food conscious. The food industry is worried, but, in general, not yet willing to undertake honest change. Rather than confronting the real problem of access to fresh, nutritious foods, the huge multinationals who control North America's food supply have made only cosmetic changes which enhance the bottom line. In the name of convenience, shelves and refrigerator displays contain synthetic foods with little nutritive value, and products removed in character and quality from the original food they are purported to contain. Add to this multiple layers of non-biodegradable packaging, bright artificial colors, and endless advertising to convince us we prefer processed and refined foods, and we see how eating becomes a political act. If the ceaseless drum of advertising were stilled, what would we want?

The miraculous rise of oat bran is an amusing example. The first question is why it is removed from oats in the first place? Bran is a natural ingredient of grains and it's good for you. Remember old-fashioned oatmeal porridge? As a granddaughter of a tall, handsome Scot I was fed a "plate" of oatmeal every morning until I went away to university. Oatmeal "stuck to the ribs," was inexpensive and quickly prepared. Then, half a century later, someone discovered that its hulls, which is what bran is, could be separated from the oat kernel and fed to humans.

After the first wave of publicity, oat bran was in dramatically short supply. It had been in bulk food stores for about the same price as wheat bran. Two weeks later it sold for five times as much—if the store could keep it in stock. "We may have to trade this under the counter," a clerk told me. Soon there were shelves and shelves of goodies—cookies, cereals, snacks, pizza, pasta, pretzels and candy bars—chock full of oat bran. Well, really! Even a good thing can be taken to unreasonable levels. As a coda on this oat bran orgy, it appears to have returned to its status as an ingredient in muffins and high-priced prepared cereals, but is still refined out of regular oats. Why do we feel so threatened, so insecure, that we grab at any straw? It is not our food that needs refining, it is us. Just last week some researchers announced that coffee is good for us after all, and that "caffeine-free" coffee is dangerous! What's next? Common sense is as important an ingredient in diet as everything else.

In our consumer age, food is one item that requires constant renewal—it is something we buy regularly. Driven by a few worldwide mega-companies, countless products are set temptingly before a gullible, affluent public. The same practices generate tragedy as millions of undernourished infants are made dependent on commercial formula. High-profile ads for this product prey on the deep desire of every woman to provide her child with "the best." The underlying message here is that mother's milk is not good enough to feed the child and that women themselves are inadequate.

Many consumers distinguish between "food" and "nutrition," food being that which tastes good, while nutrition is good for you but not much fun. So ingrained is this perception that many old-school food-industry executives still believe the worst thing that can be said about a product is that it is good for you. When you read the food pages, it may seem just about everything causes cancer or heart disease. Experts seem constantly to be changing their minds—so why bother at all? Because, in this particularly fortunate part of the world, many of us have the freedom to choose what we eat and the common sense to assist our choices.

Surely we Age Mates, with lifetimes of experience nourishing families through Depression, wartime shortages, rationing and so on, have enough smarts to see through phoney claims. We can make a difference at the checkout counter. Resolve to eat lower on the food chain. Buy non-packaged bulk foods whenever possible. These stocks usually change faster than packaged goods, the food is fresher, the unit price lower. If we think to bring our own plastic bags, layers of wasteful packaging are eliminated. And we can purchase the quantity we need without having food sitting around getting rancid. (I recently discovered a package of pudding with a coupon that had expired three years ago!) Eating lower on the food chain costs less, cuts down on fats and additives, and acknowledges the world's overall need for food while eliminating garbage.

For the last few years the public has been discovering diet as a means of preventing illness. Remember the definition of health—not just the absence of disease, but a positive state of well-being. We are entering an era of food-for-thought, recognizing that we can assist ourselves to optimum health by eating more sensibly. That means more whole grains, less meat and a wider array of fresh vegetables. Organic gardening is gaining acceptance because it minimizes the dangers of biocides in the food we eat. Organic producers are struggling to keep up with the demand even though we must sometimes accept small blemishes, pay somewhat higher prices and listen to dire warnings of economic ruin from the chemical industry.

However mixed our dietary messages have become, the confusion itself points toward change. The heavy attention seems finally to have signaled the connections between good health and pure food. For far too long such wisdom was considered off the wall. For a while only "granola people" and aging hippies insisted on pure foods grown organically. Now some of us are wondering that if we are what we eat, what does eating junk food make us?

After ignoring or ridiculing requests for information on the relationship of diet to health, some of the medical establishment appears to be moving into disease prevention through the back door. There is growing recognition of the importance of lifestyle to staying healthy, including intelligent diet. Don't miss *Diet for a New America* by John Robbins, and Frances Moore Lappé's stunning invitation to new thinking in her tenth anniversary rewrite of *Diet for a Small Planet*.

In the absence of serious attention to dietary matters by the establishment, much of the disease/diet information currently available has been collected by concerned citizens—support groups born of the need to help themselves and others. A good deal of credit goes to members of voluntary organizations like the Cancer Society, Heart Foundation and Diabetic Association, who have researched and compiled information on how to deal most effectively with their special needs. A lot of the hard work of such groups is done by Age Mates who volunteer time and expertise to compile the information we all need to make reasonable choices.

Official research results are finally coming to light, reinforcing what these support groups have suspected all along. The findings of all three special-interest groups tend to match, suggesting that the diseases of aging can be dramatically influenced by better diet. I doubt if any of the dedicated volunteer researchers think of themselves as citizen scientists, but they have opened up important areas of understanding in the prevention and treatment of chronic diseases, of concern to themselves and those they love.

Local health department dietitians can be a helpful source of information on disease prevention and up-to-date findings on the diseases of aging, both in general and as they apply specifically to women. Early nutritional information set out the desired food intake for men engaged in heavy physical labor. Women were allotted a percentage of male needs, which failed to realize women's special requirements such as additional iron and calcium. Nutritional advice continues to change as we learn more, but today's focus is on preventing or delaying major chronic degenerative diseases.

We require fewer calories as we grow older. Some of us lose the ability to digest rich foods. Always select foods with minimal processing and refining. The closer we come to eating the real thing without additives, cosmetics, fancy processing and all the other technical fixes, the healthier we are. Locally grown foods have higher vitamin content and use fewer resources than foods trucked thousands of miles. The most nutritious vegetables are the ones we grow ourselves. If each of us grew only four tomato plants in a window box or on a balcony, we could expect to harvest a good number of delicious, fresh tomatoes from each plant. Four plants multiplied by the number of Age Mates in North America would eliminate the need for a convoy of refrigerated transport trucks.

From the magic of gardening—the exercise, the anticipation and the joy of it—we will gain our very best nutrition for the spirit as well as the body. A garden is a step toward self-sufficiency and a tiny step toward solving problems for others.

Remember when we were kids we were told to eat things we didn't like to save the starving children in China or India or Africa? I tried hard to figure out how to accomplish this feat, which I would have done gladly. I would even have eaten fried cornmeal mush every day if it would have helped those starving children. In my childish opinion fried cornmeal mush was at the very bottom of the culinary barrel. It looked weird, tasted gritty and it never did make my hair curly!

But there is a way the food you don't eat can reach those who need it. When North Americans consume less red meat, land and grains are liberated for other uses. Money saved, even a little bit, can be donated to groups working to improve the lot of the world's women, who in turn can feed their children better. I do that through a non-profit organization called MATCH, as mentioned in chapter 10. There are others, but MATCH is the one I know that specifically helps women in the Third World.

We know about love and food, about preparing favorite dishes, about withholding food as punishment, being sent to bed without dinner. We know about family favoritism—giving the best bits to a favorite child, the largest portion to the dominant person and so on. Anything so fundamental as food is almost sure to be used to manipulate and control. Examples run through literature from Dickens' *Oliver Twist* to Atwood's *The Handmaid's Tale*. Institutions take advantage of this universal need by serving substandard foods to inmates or lacing meals with additives to control this or that transgression. Let it not be part of our lives.

Sometimes we don't eat properly—out of ignorance, because we are in too much of a hurry, because we are lonely, or because it doesn't seem worthwhile to go to the trouble of preparing a balanced meal for just one. Low marks for all these excuses. Take care of *you*. We have reached the time of life to show self-love through the selection and preparation of foods that respect our own needs. If you happen to be domestically challenged, inquire about a group that delivers food to your residence daily or several times a week. In some places it is called Meals on Wheels, brought to you by people ready to help.

Like everyone else, Age Mates require food for living, for fuel to go on, but for a less energetic lifestyle. In the years ahead we will experience significant changes in our living arrangements. Children leave, we move away from friends and family, purchasing power may decrease, a spouse or best friend may die, and we are deeply changed. It will affect how and what we eat. Skipping meals, eating standing up staring out the window and rushing through meals are all hard on the digestive system. Wellness is important to the enjoyment of life, and wellness requires a sensible, thoughtful diet.

What seems to lie at the center of many women's never-ending addictions to diets, is self-respect. We need to feel good about ourselves, be content with our bodies. North American women, many surrounded by every luxury and abundance, rarely believe themselves to be sufficiently attractive. Our very body may seem defective, less than perfect. Thin is said to be "in," but why? Other eras, and not too distant ones at that, valued the pleasingly plump and considered them beautiful. In other cultures a plump woman is much admired, evidence of the family's affluence.

> I made a decision to be a reasonably happy, Rubenesque
> grandmother, not a cranky, skinny one. I don't want
> rednecks to whistle at me any more.   —Age Mate, 59

Honor your body, exercise your mind and think of others as you take in nourishment. Adorn your mealtime with a flower, a candle and pleasant music. Share your meal with a friend. On special occasions, like birthdays or the full moon, why not resurrect that pleasant old fashioned custom—the potluck meal. Women make wonderful food for each other, and we never fail to come up with interesting ways of treating simple things. Age Mates no longer need to show off as we once thought we should. It is also enjoyable to cook up a pot of something in a reasonable quantity. Most of us have raised a flock of hungry kids, and only with difficulty scale down our culinary skills to meals for one or two. So make a big batch and freeze it in appropriate servings. Don't let your diet become monotonous. We can find ideas from cookbooks at the library, and from friends or our own imagination. It would be worthwhile to compile a good selection of one-person recipes in a cookbook of our own.

We have to make room in our lives for ceremony. Make your meal a sacrament. Set the table and sit down to eat. Take that time to relax, to consider your food and where it came from, and stop eating before you are full. Food is love, a gift from the planet.

Saying grace once set the scene for thoughtful relaxation, although it was sometimes difficult to be patient. My Scottish grandfather presided over meals when I was a child. Morning, noon or night until he was ninety-six, the mealtime ritual began as he reverently bowed his head, one hand to his brow, and uttered an unchanging collection of sibilants whistled through ill-fitting teeth. It calmed us five boisterous kids and the worried parents. Indigestion was unheard of. Except for the phrase "Give us this day our daily bread," we never did know what he actually said. But we believed him.

CHAPTER 13

THE MEMORY OF...

The shadowy fear of failing memory hovers over most of us. Age Mates prefer not to speak about it except in half-jesting tones. It does seem to be a legitimate worry, but like most aspects of aging, memory loss is surrounded by ignorance and misinformation, snatched from ancient baggage.

The minute we forget where we left our keys, the fear flits by on nasty little wings of doubt. Worry reinforces the concern and takes us one step closer to manifesting the fear. So think positively. To be honest with ourselves, have we not forgotten where we put the keys for decades past?

Memory is another of life's miracles. We remember millions of separate items every day—our language, how to read, how to cook, how to care for ourselves and others, smells, colors, species, mechanical skills, how to drive and routes to follow, and the bittersweet memories of things gone by. Older people remember meaningful events with utmost clarity. We may not do as well on research exercises or tests that use nonsense syllables or useless bits of measurable trivia. But why should we? Nonsense testing is of very little value to us and makes no sense to a person with six decades remembering life's experience.

The secret of most memory techniques is organizing small

pieces of material into larger groups, giving the items an understandable context. Familiarity and meaning create memorability. Memorizing by rote, the way we learned our multiplication tables, is the least useful method for committing information to long-term memory. I remember a college bout with Standard Deviation. (Standard Deviation is something done with statistics, not a personality disorder.) It seemed a meaningless mess, but the professor insisted on a passing grade. So I went into a kind of study trance for twelve straight hours, hiked off to school, passed the examination, came home, took a nap, and promptly forgot everything. Thank goodness someone invented calculators before such mathematical manipulations became important to my life.

Unless we are truly ill, we are only as forgetful as we allow ourselves to be. Memory, like the body, needs exercise. Making information rich and elaborate is one of the finest ways to intellectually stimulate yourself. The mind needs stimulation to stay sharp just as the heart needs exercise to stay strong. Most of the time the memory loss process can be reversed, but if you don't start now, your memory won't get any better. A recent long-term study of Alzheimer's concludes that the higher one's level of education and ongoing interest in learning, the less likely is the appearance of the disease. And most important to us, the researchers found that going back to school, taking night courses and participating in study groups may actually be a preventative. That's why we all rush off to study this or that at the local college. To paraphrase Louis Pasteur, chance favors the prepared mind.

Partly because of media attention, Alzheimer's may be leading us to unnecessary worry over signs of forgetfulness. What was once called senility is gradually being replaced by Alzheimer's as a focus for our concerns. Dr. Robin West, psychologist and author of *Memory Fitness over Forty* writes:

As we grow older, we do experience a definite decline in our powers of attention and concentration, two very important memory tools. On the other hand, the rate at which we forget things we've already learned does not change with age. Given the use of good techniques, practice, and daily mental stimulation, there's no reason why you can't improve your memory by 50 percent.

It may take longer these days to retrieve names, dates and phone numbers than it used to. Here memory resembles the computer, which takes nearly three times as long to find a sentence in a sixty-page file as it does in a twenty-page file. Hundreds more details are filed in our memory banks now than when we had less experience, less exposure to the world. It is not unreasonable to expect our brains to take more time to sort through mind files. Also we know more about things. Think how easy it once was to define concepts—democracy, for example. I would have given an immediate answer at sixteen, but now it would require minutes, several sentences and numerous dependent clauses. The problem here is that we are smart as well as old and have more memory, not less.

When names or dates fail to come immediately to mind we become frustrated, embarrassed or angry with ourselves and begin to think we might be in the first stages of senility or, dare we say it, Alzheimer's. What we most often notice is memory lapse, not memory loss. Think of the tens of thousands of things we *do* remember! Someone figured that if scientists could build a computer to equal the data-processing capacity of the human brain, it would require a building as big as Texas and a hundred feet high, just to enter all the permutations and combinations an ordinary human brain processes automatically. So where *did* I leave my keys? And my glasses?

Senility has no real meaning. It is a catch-all term for any episode of forgetfulness experienced by an older person. Until recently physicians assumed that senility was an inevitable part of old age, an assumption which kept them from identifying and treating true memory disorders. According to many studies, less than ten percent of our aging population—roughly the same percentage as those in nursing homes—suffer from true senile dementia, which is characterized by confusion, forgetfulness, disorientation and the inability to perform simple tasks.

For the remaining ninety-plus percent of us, three basic causes of memory loss need to be examined: physical problems, drug ingestion and nutrition. Something can be done about all three. In the majority of cases the symptoms can be traced to real, but undiagnosed, *physical problems*. Among the organic causes are anemia, constipation, hormonal imbalance, infections, urinary retention and hepatitis, all conditions which respond to medical or dietary treatment.

As discussed in Chapter 9, many Age Mates take several *prescription drugs* at the same time! The brain is very vulnerable to drug interactions, which can produce symptoms similar to those of dementia. As well as the drugs given to ambulatory patients, the additional hazard of over-medication in care facilities must not be overlooked. There the drugs prescribed often appear to benefit the staff more than the residents. The employees may be untrained or inexperienced, and are almost always seriously overworked. Many of them are recent immigrants willing to work for the pittance they are paid. They may not be able to raise questions about patient medications because of imperfect command of the language and the fear of losing their jobs or even being deported. Care facilities tend to employ the fewest possible staff members, as inexpensively as possible. Doped patients are usually malleable and quiet.

Instead of focusing high anxiety on recreational drugs like marijuana and hashish, society might be well served to look at the use of medicinal drugs, both prescribed and over-the-counter. Longtime use of mood-altering drugs may cause the appearance of senility and prolong the need for full-time care. The quality of North American life would be significantly enhanced by a more intelligent use of prescription drugs.

Among people who are aging poorly, a third area to examine is *eating habits*. You don't have to have a terrible diet to suffer nutritional deficiency. It may seem like a lot of trouble to prepare proper meals for yourself, but a little time and effort expended to assure nutritious food is significantly less of a problem in the long run than developing full-blown memory loss. Take your vitamins and eat balanced meals. Then try to remember where you left your keys.

A number of specific disorders can lead to memory loss and confusion. *Most of them are reversible and should be identified and treated.* Correct diagnosis is extremely important. The mental symptoms of these diseases often resemble those of Alzheimer's, and they may cause misdiagnosis or be dismissed as senility.

Watch out for DBL!

DBL stands for Depression, Boredom and Loneliness, states of mind that accompany or feed on each other. These threaten to destroy morale and send you into a downward spiral. Catch them early before they catch you. This is a good time to enlist the help of Age Mate friends.

Mental depression is probably the disorder most commonly misdiagnosed, especially when low self-esteem forms part of the picture. Depression is often socially inflicted. Too often we fall prey to the unrealistic demand that all women live up to an imagined stereotype. Society's inability to accept normal aging is the real disease and cries out for responsible therapy. Meanwhile we are likely to be caught up in feelings of worthlessness, forfeiting the possibilities of dynamic, productive lives. The depression that follows may result in a slowing of speech and movement, slowing of thought, changes in sleep and eating habits, decreased pleasure in any sort of activity, and underestimating one's true abilities. Drugs and alcohol affect mood, memory and speed of reactions. Alcohol can worsen depression. Failure to recognize the part depression plays in aging causes public and personal attention to focus on the wrong things.

Samuel Johnson said that the art of memory is the art of attention. When we can't remember a piece of information, it may be that we never really paid attention to it in the first place. Since we didn't encode it firmly in memory, it's no surprise that it's not there when we go to look for it. Back to the computer model, unless you consciously "save" every bite you punch in, you'll *never* find it again. I lost one whole chapter in this book that way, and it had to be rewritten from the beginning. (It was, by coincidence, Chapter 13!)

We run much of our lives on automatic pilot. The longer we live, of course, the more time we spend on habitual behavior patterns. We repeat our maintenance schedules so often that they can be performed without thinking. When we are on automatic pilot we rarely take special note, and hence specific happenings fail to sink in. When we do things in a different way, and we pay attention to what is happening *now*—we read anew the signs, the actions, body language, and note that which is relevant to the new experience.

About teaching an old dog new tricks, it is now widely accepted that one retains the ability to learn throughout one's lifetime. Recent research studies at Wichita State University in Kansas discovered that people sixty and older are excellent students. Among faculty members whose classes were audited, more than 75 percent said their over-sixty students were at least as quick to learn as younger ones and 64 percent reported they seemed more motivated. Three out of five faculty members said the mature students made a positive difference in their classes.

One learns when surrounded by learning opportunities. More than half the older students attended campus events, read the college newspaper and regularly used school facilities such as the student centre, and particularly the library. Not only did they feel they benefited from the learning, but they enjoyed the people on campus even more than the classes. When your memory needs a tune-up, enroll in a class or audit a course that interests you, and enjoy the side effects.

There are some simple techniques to help remember things. If you are worried about forgetting someone, make a nonsense rhyme out of the name, fasten on some distinctive feature of a face, fix the first letter in your mind. "Just a minute. The name begins with B." Or ask the person to spell the name. I did that once and the name turned out to be S-m-i-t-h. Oh well, sometimes we goof! I haven't forgotten it though.

My partner takes note of names by figuring out how they sound backwards. He is fabulous with crosswords and unbeatable at *Trivial Pursuit.* You may find that turning information into sayings, rhymes and images can be quite an entertaining way of remembering. Decorate an event or number with some outlandish imagining for easy recall.

Develop your own ways to remember to do a task, pay a bill, keep an appointment. I slip a ring from one hand to the other and tell myself firmly why I put it there. I've been doing that for fifty years. Sometimes going to the place where a thought first crossed your mind will help recall it. Make a list every day that includes the things you want to remember to do. When my list includes huge things like Finish Book, or Make a Will, I pad my list with things like Wash Dishes, Put out the Garbage, Brush the Cats—so there are some things to cross off! Crossing things off a list is one of life's pleasures, as well as a memory exercise. Transferring them to a list day after day is not such a pleasure!

Like mislaid treasures, memories may reappear from nowhere. Sometimes a memory from long ago just arrives in your consciousness. It may be the sight of a particular color or pattern, or a tune long forgotten. One source of memory is the sense of smell. Encoding odors takes place in the brain's most primitive section, the limbic brain. It is the first part to develop in the embryo, and apparently remains a major source of identification in all creatures. Mothers recognize their newborn infants by smell as well as sight; birds return to breeding grounds following odors. Watch dogs and cats sniff at strangers to decide whether or not certain people are friendly. It is also said that we humans can smell fear, tension, hostility. Fish are thought to follow mysterious scents in the rivers of their birth, to bring them safely home to spawn. I wonder which stream they follow when spawned in fish hatcheries?

Olfactory centers contain a treasury of memory. Whenever I smell a certain kind of chewing gum, a beloved friend from sixty years ago rises strong and tall in my mind's eye. The scent of moss and fir needles brings me back to the edge of a forest in my home town. Autumn leaves and ocean breezes carry memories, as does the smell of new books and, for me, especially crayons. I visited a crayon factory once and was overwhelmed by nostalgia.

Although our society does its best to eliminate personal scents with deodorants, sprays and cleaning compounds, we may be deliberately confusing our memories and stopping ourselves from recognizing pleasures and dangers that odors normally signal. When the ability to smell becomes impaired, we lose something of the spice of life, as well as diminishing clues to memories.

Like all valuable possessions, memory must be cared for. Rather than letting it slip into disuse, practice keeping mental facilities in good working order. We are designed to live not only long, but fully.

For years I have been dismayed when brilliant ideas flit across my mind and vanish in thin air. They glow for an instant like phosphorescence in the sea and just as mysteriously disappear. I'm dispirited when bright ideas appear at inconvenient times, when it's too late or I'm too tired to write them down. I'm sorry when they are only a faint memory in the morning. Many of us share this experience.

Years ago a very special twenty-year-old insisted that thoughts will come back when they are needed. He advised me not to fret about it, but trust that the right ideas will come at the right time. "Nothing," he said, "is ever lost, and nothing is unimportant." It sounded mystical, and in a life of stress and competitiveness, I didn't think the lad made sense. He, and many philosophers I have since consulted, say the same thing—nothing is ever wasted, nothing is an accident, and everything begins with a thought— maybe even the universe itself is God's thought.

Buddhist philosophy bids adherents to follow the Eightfold Path of Right Living, and theorizes that when one proceeds from "right" motives, everything has a purpose and will be available when circumstances are right. The whole fabulous idea, eerie though it seems, has hung around the corners of my mind for decades. It would be so agreeable—just to trust in your own wisdom, act from the right motives and believe the "right" skills and thoughts will emerge from somewhere to assist in the manifestation of what you rightly desire to bring into being.

After these many years, I now think that once-strange notion may be true. Thoughts, like memories, sometimes arrive from nowhere just when they are needed. Pay special attention to coincidences. Sometimes a book falls open to display an important idea. A conversation is overheard and supplies the notion that had eluded weeks of thought. The title for this book arrived that way. Sometimes important matters become clear from an unexpected encounter, or a grand idea sweeps in from a dream, unbidden, its origins unknown. I dreamed we should hold a gathering of older women to get acquainted with our power and reinforce the many qualities we share. In time this dream became The Amazing Grays. The mysterious capacity to access information is part of each person's storehouse of karma. It seems the more one holds oneself open toward life and the universe, while approaching each day with a sense of faith and trust, the more will guidance and intuition become available. That is probably where the good medicine is stored.

We can choose what we want to remember. It is even possible

to give yourself a happy childhood by remembering events and activities that were pleasant, weeding out the old hurts and might-have-beens. It doesn't always work, but by using creative visualization it is possible to surround ugliness in a mental bubble and blow it away, leaving memory space for moments of wonder and tenderness that are there for your recall. Exorcise the ghosts. Tell them to go away. Bring the good memories forward into the light, clear out the shadows, consign the uglies to the twilight zone, and let the light of loving memory shine around you. Make it your intention to let your life reflect reverence in all you do, and this includes a reverence for your life as well as life in the universe.

My friend Mildred Tremblay brought a poem to a writing class we were taking. She spoke the memories of her woman's body, a memory we so often repress. As I felt the warmth of her words, a whole flood of memory encompassed me. The glory of being a female person, rich in experience and love, surrounded me. Remembering, I asked her to share it with you.

> In those days
> my breasts and belly
> like a field, perhaps
> plowed by the moon
> I was nature's favorite
> I teemed with cycles
> I waxed and waned
> I swarmed with life
>   oh it was splendid
> I cast off the egg
> I held the egg
> birth raged through me
> I arched I heaved I panted
> I screamed beautifully
> my body was a river

down which the blind babes
turned and twisted
lost their way
found it again
It seems my belly
was always sore
or tender or cramped
I was swollen or stretched
or bloody or torn
    oh it was splendid
my breasts weighted
my nipples powerful
tough and brown
shaped to the pull
    of sucking mouths
crusted with cream
sweet milk leaking
I was like a garden
tilled dug seeded
I blossomed
I was always blossoming
    now it is over
    I am quiet

CHAPTER 14

THE ADVENTURE OF SEX

Sex? Yes, it's always there, but it's not the big ticket item it used to be.
                                                    —Age Mate, 72

Well, here we are! I never imagined that someday long after menopause, I would belong to the ranks of sexually active seniors. In fact, like many of my generation, when I was much younger I spent a certain amount of time speculating on whether my parents managed this most intimate of all relationships. With five kids in the family I knew it had to happen sometimes, but as a general thing it seemed quite remote. Of course my grandparents *never* did such a thing. Now, here I am with my oldest granddaughter about to graduate from university. I wonder if she is wondering about me! I recall the story of one little boy who asked where babies came from, as children often do. His father gave him a careful description of the process, and the youngster looked him right in the eye and declared, "Not me!"

When it comes to sexuality you must *not* believe anyone under sixty! The rumor that sexual activity stops at forty-five or any arbitrary age is simply untrue. Pay no attention to rumors and false prophets. Sex after sixty is much like any other activity—you get back what you put into it.

Instead of writing your sexual obituary, be prepared for surprises, possibly even miracles. In this age of possibilities, new, compassionate relationships are free to develop based on love and understanding. We are largely excused from singles bars and one-night stands, and not many of us would want to return. The fundamentals of "elder sex" are shared memories and warm familiarity. At last women no longer need fear pregnancy, and men are free from any need to demonstrate machismo.

Sexuality *is* always there. It may change in superficial ways, but for women, at least, this fundamental aspect of being human has the possibility of becoming more satisfying and more fulfilling as time goes by. Despite myths to the contrary, most women retain active interest in loving sex long past menopause. This is such a remarkable thought that several otherwise intelligent books on aging hardly mention sex at all. Perhaps it is the notion that sexual activity consists only of intercourse that is at fault. That definition is most often the product of male assumption, without benefit of women's point of view. The need to give and receive loving tenderness is never lost. It remains forever a bond between life partners, and can form the basis of new relationships. The notion that sexuality disappears with age is incorrect.

For the most part, intelligent discussion of sex among older people is still largely taboo. From personal experience and my own research, I conclude that just as we know very little about the physiology of normal menopause, so too do we know little about the attitudes and preferences of the sexually active postmenopausal woman. Again, much of the information comes from a medical profession which sees mainly sick or impaired women, assumes they are asexual, and generally approaches ageful women as ailing women. Progressive practitioners admit they have a limited knowledge about healthy aging. I have found little printed information about the extraordinary changes under-gone by our half of the human population, let alone information about our sexuality.

> The mind of a post-menopausal woman is virtually
> uncharted territory, for men have shown little inclination to
> explore it. Doctors and psychiatrists glibly ascribe any or all
> of her difficulties to "menopausal depression," or a similar
> diagnostic catchall. However, it may be that her real needs
> and urges simply are not understood, so the experts have no
> jargon to describe them, just as our society has no symbol to
> represent them.   —Barbara G. Walker, *The Crone*

It's about as difficult now to learn about mature sexuality as it was to find an unexpurgated copy of *Fanny Hill* in our youth. The truth seems to be that after the end of their fertile time, the large majority of women (and their partners) discover whole new realms of sexual pleasure, as well as what several women told me is a "new lease on life."

Age changes the nature of sexual expression from rambunctious power trips to a more tender, caring, even romantic focus on relationships. After menopause there may be a great blossoming of sexuality as we let our inhibitions go. It is all right to become sexual!

Far from being a disease or curse, *menopause is liberating!* No one told us *this!* The general surge of energy and sense of well-being that follows menopause will find most of us intellectually and physically more active, more involved and often much happier. It is a remarkable time of change when we begin to do things differently than we were expected to do in our child-rearing years. Barbara Walker, in *The Crone*, puts it this way:

> We hear much about women's nest-building instincts,
> which, after all, form the economic foundation of our

consumer society; but we hear little of any nest-destroying behavior, which may be equally instinctive. . . .

An older woman may experience strong urges to weed out her possessions, to simplify her life by purging it of excessive impedimenta, to move to smaller quarters and keep them neater, to restrict her social contacts to a few good friends instead of a wide circle of acquaintances. She may give things away, neglect her house, stop buying clothes. If she is still acquisitive, it may be only in respect to a personal enthusiasm, such as a collection, unrelated to the interests of other family members.

Behavioral changes like these come as quite a shock to traditional males who expect their women to continue their nurturing role forever. One of the least-tolerated changes in the older woman's behavior is her withdrawal from the other-directed activity of her mothering years. Men apparently expect women to wait on them, satisfy their whims, abet their acquisitiveness, support their efforts and carry on as titillating sex objects, while the men continue to strive for advancement. Middle-aged men who seek to increase their power and community stature for as long as possible, require obliging wives to be successful. They often expect ongoing caretaking, with or without realizing the wife might have her own needs. In our society, men are conditioned to keep control over women, and as their sexual potency declines, many men go to extremes to maintain that control. This may explain reports that wife-beating frequently takes place immediately after sexual intercourse.

There is evidence to suggest that mature women would enjoy more, rather than less, sexual activity. Not necessarily so with males. Regrettably, our society focuses much attention on the deteriorating sexual desirability of women, but little on similar deterioration in males. Probably all of us have heard derogatory assessments of the old woman's "slack vagina," but very little is said about the decreased turgidity of the aging penis. In a nutshell, a penis that has enjoyed sixty-plus years of service eventually shows the wear. If male or female were any sort of machine, sixty years of friction would erode mortar *and* pestle beyond recognition. A remarkable instrument, the human body, with its powers of maintenance and regeneration.

Signs of wear begin in most males somewhere in the fourth or fifth decade. Unfortunately, men tend to express worry about their decreasing sexual vigor by fixing on unfounded assumptions about *female* sexuality. It has long been customary for the male to blame the female for any malfunction of his own, and the sexual changes wrought by aging are no exception. Fantasies of rejuvenation arising from an endless procession of nubile maidens may or may not be effective, but it's certain that no one askes the maidens their opinion on the subject.

While we were producing the Baby Boom of the forties and fifties, there were jokes among doctors in which the gynecologist was told to "take another stitch for me" while sewing up the then-standard episiotomy. In anticipation of a loose vagina, men hoped to "make as much use of the equipment as possible before the warranty ran out." Such degrading sexist outlooks have, I hope, ceased in this more enlightened era.

The whole macho thing is a cruel habit designed to increase women's feelings of inadequacy, sexual and otherwise. The notion that mature female genitalia are unresponsive is false. What would help more women and men achieve sexual fulfillment at any age is a less biased examination of the mythology surrounding the omnipotent male organ. Things change. The over-sixty-year-old penis can no longer anticipate the triumph of the macho limerick which concludes "he punctured a mattress, two sheets and an actress, and shattered a bedroom utensil." Nor can Mr. Big expect to hold up his end, as per another joke, under several slices of salami, mustard and a pickle. The punchline, sisters, was "It looked so good I ate it myself." *(Author's note*: If this book unfortunately lands with a male editor, it may never get published.)

We were conditioned to regard our genitalia as nasty, unclean, smelly. Certain churches even forbade young girls the delight of patent leather shoes for fear they, or the little boys they played with, would see those shameful private parts reflected in them. The pleasures of masturbation were denied us, and for many of us the shame persists. So much distortion results when prurient minds exert their influence over innocence.

While female genitalia were cursed and shamed, apparently no such restrictions cast shame on the male organ, which was displayed with pride, but only on *his* terms. Take the example of girlie magazines. Have you ever wondered why we could never catch a glimpse of any sort of penis, let alone an erect one? Why was the male organ concealed when women were shown in ever more revealing postures? Men sometimes appeared in the photographs, usually fully clothed, their faces rarely identifiable. Why, amid all this sexual display, was there never an erection in sight? Was the male not excited by the sexual perfection arranged before him? Was he demonstrating his superiority by remaining aloof from the tantalizing property? Apparently many women have fantasized about the photographer and his models, but for all the evidence of sexuality disclosed by their artistry the photographers must not have reacted in the same vein.

The double standard applied to the display of sex organs tells us erotic energy is not a matter for mutual appreciation, but one under male control. A young girl seeking information on male anatomy in these publications was about as far behind as I was with Grandma's *Doctor Book*. A pubescent female glancing through magazine display racks would be forgiven if she concluded that the penis was an invisible organ, and that the male has no balls at all.

Remember the scandals around the Kinsey Report? Remember the grimy edges of those four pages in *Gone With the Wind*? The sexy bits. And the censorship uproar over *Lady Chatterley's Lover*? We passed pirated (maybe stolen) copies of *Esquire* magazines around the girls' dorm at college. Later six girls borrowed a car and drove for hours to find a movie theater showing an uncut version of *Ecstasy*. How times change! The hunger to understand the wonderful, mysterious power of sexuality occupied us—mind and body—to the point of obsession. We knew there had to be something more than babies, more than just "satisfying a man," however that was accomplished.

I think all this secrecy stunted our sexual development. Why was it desirable to deny women knowledge of the male sex? My guess is that men either thought it was unimportant or found it difficult to endure comparison. Facing up to the possibility that his own magnificent organ might be less magnificent than those of his fellows was just too painful. Thus the publishers spared their largely male readers the need for honesty by exploiting the female in ever more degrading situations. With far too many males the penis was apparently the same as self-esteem. The language disclosed its high status: "my tool" for the working class, "my sceptre" for the nobility, "my weapon" for all.

As with aging women there is little empirical evidence on the sexuality of aging males. His sex is on display throughout his life, and he is apparently expected to brandish it boldly. When he experiences normal changes, apparently his very sense of self is threatened. He is also handicapped by the cruel myth that says he reaches his sexual peak at around seventeen, and everything goes downhill after that. Because of the extraordinary importance of masculine sexual performance, whole species of animals are being annihilated to help him retain his sexual prowess—rhinoceros horn, bear gall bladder, seal genitals, the velvet on the horns of deer, elk and moose, to mention only a few.

A great many men appear to know everything about "screwing" but very little about loving. Some men still think penis size is the crucial factor in successful lovemaking. Because men so often fail to take the woman's interests into account, concern over penis size may be just an easy way out for those who aren't willing to learn about women's real needs and sexual desires. It's not what you have, men. It's how skillfully you use it.

The older male does not have to cease being a lover because he has trouble with his erection. Nor is his inability to obtain an erection the woman's fault. When he gets past the juvenile notion of rampaging conquest, there is a whole world of sexuality awaiting discovery. There is a new realm of tenderness, gentleness and sensitivity to his *own* capacity to express love and satisfy his partner. Sexuality doesn't die; it is transformed from the frightening urgency of youth into a warm and mellow exchange of intimacy between loving partners who know and understand each other. Women want to be *willing* sexual partners with the freedom to respond honestly, or to say *no* without recriminations.

Neither are men to be disparaged for *their* changing physiology. All is normal within a loving relationship so long as one's actions are informed by kindness. What does seem to be a source of struggle is the male ego. Can he recognize the changes to *his* physiology wrought by time, and accept them? As Germaine Greer said in a radio interview many years ago, "Who said you can't have fun with a limp penis?" In fact, you don't need any kind of penis to have fun, as lesbian Age Mates have always known. Respect, tenderness and imagination are what make good sex.

When, after all life's changes, we lie warm and satisfied in the arms of a loved partner, holding memories and joys and each other, we will have achieved a state of being worth carrying into Paradise.

> If I'm supposed to die any time soon, I hope it happens while we're making love—if I wouldn't ruin everything for my partner.
> —Age Mate, 59

Most of us were well into or beyond our childbearing years before the "new morality" came in view. We missed the sexual revolution. That's the bad news. The good news is that in our maturity we have the freedom to experience our sexuality fully, creatively, with the wisdom and compassion of our years.

Now that it is all right for the woman to initiate sex, we have permission to woo our partners. You may need to drag a tired, reluctant lover to your private party, but he'll be glad he came once you convince him. Statistics, for what they are worth, say that men, too, change their appreciation of sexuality as they mature. Due to sheer physiological limitations, most will pass beyond the heavy, macho, conquering phase and will no longer need to show off their sexual prowess, which, according to women willing to discuss the matter, wasn't always that great anyway.

Our cultural emphasis on the orgasm as the be-all and end-all of sexuality is a pity. By focusing only on orgasm, both partners are deprived of playfulness, loving consideration of each other, and the gentleness that is so important to sexual expression. The importance of foreplay went unrecognized in the era of "wham, bam, thank you ma'am." Once the female orgasm was discovered it turned a number of participating females into actresses. Faking an orgasm is among the tricks of most women's trade. For a wonderful laugh, see the film, *When Harry Met Sally*. Harry's conviction that a woman could not fake an orgasm was embarrassingly shaken while he and Sally were dining at a sedate restaurant.

Sex that was supposed to be so great often wasn't. There *had* to be something more! What we got was titillating, inaccurate stuff to nourish the tide of awakening sexuality. Many of us didn't really find out what was missing until our Baby Boom daughters spelled it out for us decades later.

They hung our version of sex and sexual attractiveness in the closet and came out with joyful, unspeakable things like letting their hair hang down without curlers, hair spray, or adornments thought to entice males. No makeup! No bra! They didn't know what a girdle was. They didn't even shave their legs! Nor was there a sexy piece of clothing anywhere in the backpack. They wore shapeless shirts, patched and wrinkled jeans. My daughter didn't iron anything except her hair for five years.

And *then* there was premarital sex! Living together without benefit of clergy or the fluffy white wedding dress. No worry about "till death do us part." Our daughters announced theirs was the new morality and "women's lib." Often we mothers couldn't understand. The behavioral changes we tried to comprehend were both sociological and sexual. These liberated daughters were not going to suppress *their* natural selves because of silly old rules that weren't important anyway. "Look at you and Dad. I'm not going to be like *you*!"

That there might be long-range complications other than pregnancy went largely unrecognized. We didn't know about AIDS in those days. The most common sexually transmitted diseases were kept in check with antibiotics, and the Pill eliminated worry about pregnancies. Whether they were straight or gay, our sons and daughters displayed their flamboyant sexuality in beads and bright colors, racy music and catchy slogans—"make love, not war." Many parents were shaken as society swung a hundred and eighty degrees around them.

It was traumatic. Confusing. Painful. We *didn't* understand. Our own carefully raised kids behaving in ways we could scarcely believe! Many a tear-filled day, many a sleepless night passed in worry and heartbreak when they went far from us in their rebellion. When they came back, and most of them did, they returned with more knowledge and information than their parents or their lagging schools could possibly teach them. They had seen the world. Painful though it seemed at the time, when they did come home—probably stoned—they were far more humane than when they left, more open, less uptight, less judgmental except where parents were concerned.

The young people I knew overflowed with altruism. It was at this time that the US Peace Corps flowered, and the Company of Young Canadians reached out around the world to return with an international perspective which is one of our best hopes for making our world as good as it can be. Their dynamic ideas were at least partly the result of the new morality. Previous generations had used much of their idealistic energy to repress sexuality and keep it under socially sanctioned control.

While our children, boys and girls, launched themselves happily into the whirlpool of sexuality, we could only look on in a mixture of rejection and envy. Their apparent delight was denied us in our time. Stern morality was part of it, as was our readiness for husbands to dominate.

When we were young, we did not think human reproduction could be under our control. Most of our reproductive years went by before the invention of the Pill. We were taught restraint, refusal and denial as the only ways to deal with our sexuality in the rare instances when the matter was discussed. In some places we could not be fitted with a contraceptive diaphragm unless we were married, and sometimes such a fitting required the husband's consent. *No* was often the final word in male/female conversations. The Victorian-reared women who mothered so many of us had a frightening view of man's "animal nature." Woman's responsibility was to put the brakes on before marriage and to "do her duty" after marriage, whether she wished to or not. Marriage among the elite in those days might be partly for pleasure, partly for status, but mostly it was about making a "good catch" who would take care of us. Of those of us who were lesbians, few dared to say so.

Our generation of women inherited many of those narrow views. In the absence of anything more informative than *Marjorie May's Twelfth Birthday* (a pamphlet put out by a manufacturer of sanitary pads just beginning to run discreet magazine ads), small-town

America was without much information. We went to extraordinary lengths to conceal menstruation and probably still would. Some girls actually didn't know where babies came from, let alone how they got there. The library in my town had a locked room for books that included mention of "IT" or for any explicit novels that had slipped through the library censors. What we learned about physiology was either by accident, like seeing a baby brother's penis, or from the most authentic of all sources, *The Doctor Book.*

Whatever bothered you, from "the vapors" to venereal disease was in *The Doctor Book*. It contained enlightening, colored, fold-together models of the human body. My grandmother's 1905 edition, which I recently inherited, has hand-painted illustrations of blood vessels, lungs, intestines and all those good things. However, it didn't tell me what I really wanted to know. Grandma had torn off "all the naughty bits" and kept them in a separate envelope, which I never did find.

Our generation was too often taught that sex was disgusting, nasty or bad. It was restricted by the Church, warned against by mothers and relegated to hushed, forbidden discussions. It's small wonder that we were often unable to understand our own sexuality even as hormones raced recklessly through our maturing bodies. Girls who "went all the way" were "cheap" and scared. Boys wouldn't respect us. At the very least we expected to get pregnant or contract a horrible disease. A disfiguring disease at that. Those were the days before the discovery of antibiotics. Sulfa and penicillin would liberate society from the early effects of most sexually transmitted diseases, but not until after the war. Giving erotic pleasure to ourselves or to other women was so forbidden it was never even mentioned.

The pain and unhappiness of our suppressed sexuality still haunts many Age Mates in one way or another. So much of the negative conditioning stayed with us and filtered into our adult lives, inhibiting both ourselves and our partners. That was before women had much of a sense of themselves as independent persons. We thought of ourselves as the exclusive property of men, of husbands whom we might not meet for many years.

Although we knew having children was our destiny, the constant fear of pregnancy before marriage dominated our hunger to discover our own sexuality. The wondrous, thrilling sensations of our young bodies had to be suppressed, hidden away beneath social and moral restrictions. Men only married "nice girls," we were told, and because the possibility of being without a man was nearly unthinkable back there in the thirties and forties, we devoted a good deal of effort to staying "nice." It was said men wouldn't marry us if we were not virgins. We were unsuitable for "good" men if we gave in, even to the good men themselves. It was always the woman in her weakness who was at fault, while a snicker of approval greeted young men who sowed their wild oats, or they carved notches in their gun stocks. Fathers of lusty daughters routinely bragged about keeping their shotguns at the ready to ward off unsuitable suitors.

These experiences may not have been universal, but half a century ago they were the norm in towns and villages where the majority of us lived. In my small town a girl who got pregnant was an object of intense scorn, the subject of endless gossip, ostracized, sent away to some breeding home for wayward girls, and sometimes not allowed back into the community. Abortion for ordinary women was impossible except in a dangerous, terrifying back alley where women, especially poor women, could and did die. By then, North America had thoroughly medicalized reproduction, and the midwife who might have advised and counseled women had been drummed out of town.

There were orphanages near major centers, and rumors of "doorstep babies." Even after proper adoption, life for the infant conceived out of wedlock was often difficult. The stigma of illegitimacy frequently followed the child all its life. Yet it must have been common. I have three close friends seeking their birth mothers and in my Women's Circle, five of thirty-two women did not know their paternal grandmother's name. Perhaps we are free enough at last to validate our existence, legitimate or not. Bastards were regarded with contempt except in certain chapters of European history where they became kings and courtiers.

Adoption was the best of a number of unsatisfactory choices, but was not much comfort to the new mother who had to "put her child up" to God knows whom to be cared for God knows how. The few of our contemporaries who bucked the social norms and kept their children despite all the scorn and censure were brave indeed. An unmarried mother was a constant example to those of us who felt our sexuality, but were afraid. "You be careful, young lady, or you'll end up just like her." I can't remember any girls who kept their babies who were also allowed to return to school. The conventional morality excluded unmarried mothers from contact with other, presumably more innocent, girls. Although these restrictions may have differed from place to place, it was a pretty uptight time everywhere. It came out of the Depression, the Dust Bowl, and real poverty when about the only thing there was to hang onto was the morality of days gone by. It preserved the patriarchy at a time when the power of a failing economy and the drought had undermined male self-respect. Men could always feel powerful where daughters were concerned.

The boys went away to war as soon as they could sign up. Girls at home were held as some sort of hostage to a past that would never come again. The point was to keep the daughter desirable as a wife so she could be handed over with pride and sometimes profit. We were passed from the watchful attention of the father to the absolute control of the husband.

Sexual mores began to change when the boys came home from World War Two. The old song that went "How you gonna keep them down on the farm, after they've seen Paree?" was mostly about sex. Girls, alone in a world of fantasy and Hollywood movies, had "kept" themselves for their men through the long years. Returning servicemen, having savored less puritan moralities in Europe and Asia, expected the little girl next door to give in. When she didn't, he sought other outlets. Feeling close to death all that time gave him license to express his sexuality and released him from social censure. Both sexes went through difficult transitions, and much misunderstanding. I know one man who didn't marry the girl he loved because she wouldn't, and spent twenty unhappy years married to one who would. "Frigidity" was the word used to shame women who said no.

Premarital restrictions were bad enough, but the fear of pregnancy penetrated even marriage. An unwanted pregnancy could ruin a whole career. Abstinence, the rhythm method, the diaphragm and coitus interruptus were far from reliable means of contraception. One medical student I knew aborted his wife more than once. She cried on my shoulder. I also knew a couple where the husband had a promising future as a graduate student, but had to quit his studies when his wife got pregnant. They had only her wages to live on. When young people married in those days they were on their own. At the end of the Depression or after the maturing experience of war, few parents would or could support a young couple. Withdrawal of economic support may also have been used as punishment for expressing sexuality.

At a tenth anniversary party my neighbor, a mother of six, said it was the first anniversary that she wasn't pregnant or nursing. I knew another woman who believed she had reached menopause. She and her husband set out to celebrate, in her words, "Our first-ever uninhibited weekend," and found herself pregnant at forty-nine!

Both women and men have been cheated by the notion that intercourse is all there is to sex. The guys were supposed to be so powerful and smart, women so innocent and stupid, and neither had a reliable place to go for answers. In the 1960s, sex started screaming from every billboard. Insinuations about a hysterically wonderful, totally carefree, irresponsible sex life were all around. The home-bound, child-rearing housewife (that's our generation) felt as if she were missing something, maybe missing everything. It was a rough time, very hard on our self-respect. Women thought about their routine, usually colorless couplings and felt cheated. Husbands started looking around to deal with their own frustration. May/September pairings have been relatively common among our husbands in recent decades.

Among their secretaries, nurses and students, quite a few midlife men found charming, intelligent young women to help them see life anew. Adventurous academics and businessmen decided to change their lives by changing partners. They were often attracted to colleagues, women with budding careers, filling responsible roles. These women were independent, able to make their own decisions, and open to attention and affection. Attractive, daughter-aged women lived their lives in sharp contrast to the stay-at-home wives who still filled their roles as the culture of their youth had insisted they do. More often than one might expect, the young, exciting second loves were much like the first wives when they were younger. Lots of marriages broke up in the seventies and eighties—our marriages.

> Harold came home Friday night, put his arms around me,
> held me close and said he loved me all these thirty-seven
> years, and would always love me. He kissed me tenderly.
> And then he left.   —Age Mate, 66

We might wonder also about the young women who are now our former partners' wives and lovers. The dozen or so I know are intelligent and able, not at all like the "gold diggers" of popular myth. Is it possible that they were seeking the fathers they never knew? The busy, dedicated men who found it difficult to get home from the office, who noticeably favored sons above daughters and probably didn't think much about their girl-children except that they would just get married and give them grandchildren.

The effect of sexuality distorted by the social mores of our youth continues to ripple through our generation. It lodges in the myth of the sexless older woman whose desire was thought to vanish long before age sixty. This attitude has enabled various authorities to exercise cruel and autocratic treatment of the aged. Some nursing homes discourage any sexual contact, even to the extent of separating husbands from wives. They seem unable or unwilling to recognize elders' need for closeness, companionship and mature love. Through the ignorance of society this lovely, natural expression of human compassion between older people is turned into something disgusting and unclean. We better find out where these sorts of administrators are coming from, and send them back!

Sexuality among the aging population is very much alive, but different. Two things that change are the male's ability and the older woman's willingness to service her man regardless of her own wishes. With the achievement of age, she *can* say no. A curious corollary to this discovery are reports that the majority of males in high-pressure jobs experience some degree of impotence—and blame their old wives.

We have more or less accepted the new morality. Two New York doctor/professors surveyed over eight hundred US seniors about their sexual attitudes and activities. Ninety-seven percent like sex. Ninety-one percent approved of unmarried or widowed older people having sex or living together. Seventy-five percent think sex now feels as good as or better than it did when they were young. Seventy-two percent were satisfied with their sexual experiences, and 80 percent think that sex is good for their health. The information was collected from men and women between the ages of sixty and ninety-one.

Another survey of 100 men and 102 women aged 80 to 102 living in retirement homes (and willing to fill out a 117-item questionnaire!) reported the most common sexual activity was touching and caressing without intercourse. Masturbation was second most common, with sexual intercourse third. Seventy percent of the men and 50 percent of the women often or very often fantasized or daydreamed about intimate relations. About half felt that retirement-home living did not preclude sex, and felt that it actually increased their chances for sex at least part of the time.

Sexuality may also regenerate under certain conditions. An Age Mate of sixty-two told me she thought she had "dried up" years ago and then she met this interesting widower:

> I was surprised when I found a pleasant, rosy feeling
> building up in my loins, and my female juices flowing like a
> teenager. This is the best time of all. I'm finding out what
> sex is all about, and I don't have to worry about getting
> pregnant.

Remembering all these early traumas suggests that the Pill has probably liberated more heterosexual women than anything else. It has contributed in large measure to the rise of feminism and the women's liberation movement. It has allowed women to control their reproductive lives and enjoy the possibilities of their own bodies.

Whatever its alleged side effects, the Pill has brought peace of mind, sexual harmony and joy to women who love men. Reliable contraception has also created problems which required difficult choices. Our male-dominated society—through its lawmakers, its courts, its churches—continues to struggle with moral and ethical dilemmas surrounding reproductive technology and a woman's right to control her own body. We are still a long way from having the freedom to enjoy our sexuality, but it is a lot better than it was.

What remains in need of desperate attention is an equitable way of dealing with unwanted pregnancies. Surely a woman must not be obliged to farm her body out to produce offspring that she does not want or cannot care for. On the other hand, destroying a life desiring to be born is also wrong in the eyes of many Age Mates. Abortion is not a solution responsible women readily choose. What is clearly missing is responsible *male* parenthood. I have asked members of our Canadian Parliament to devise suitable penalties for men who impregnate women against their will. So far none of the government officials I contacted have deigned to answer. It seems to me that legislators and right-to-lifers believe in immaculate conception, assigning no responsibility to the male. Whatever our beliefs, when we older women register our opinions on this difficult question, may we do it without bitterness or recrimination, and particularly, without righteousness.

Marriage, like sexuality itself, is undergoing change. The traditional timing of events in the life cycle is altered by our longer life spans. Women and men marry, divorce, remarry and divorce again up through their seventies. In times where almost any configuration of relationships is more or less acceptable, we have choices. Today's marriages are not carved in stone. Permanence is not obligatory. Women do not have to pair up with men in order to be acceptable or fulfilled in their lives. They can become loving friends with men, and with other women, or they can choose "single blessedness." One largely unacceptable combination that continues shrouded in taboo is the younger male with the older female. The relationship tenderly explored in the movie *Harold and Maude,* and more recently in the television series *thirtysomething,* may become more acceptable, given women's longer life expectancy.

In 1990, Ann Landers published a letter from a woman who signed herself "Content in Montreal." She said she and her husband, both in their late fifties, had given up sex when they were in their forties. "We are extremely compatible, happily married and don't feel that we are missing a thing." The question she asked was, "Are we oddballs? How many other married couples live together happily without sex?" More than thirty-five thousand people wrote in.

> My mail tells me that men of all ages are far more interested in sex than women and an amazing number of women in all age groups consider sex a duty or a nuisance. They pretend to enjoy it and fake orgasms to keep their men happy. Some couples gave up on sex in their early thirties while others were still enjoying it in their eighties.
> —Ann Landers, June 26, 1990

My own research tells me women do enjoy sex and want it, but not when sex is centered on the male's pleasure. But even when both partners are committed to mutual enjoyment, the truth is that the sex act can be painful for older women. Although it is a difficult topic for many of us to discuss, vaginal secretions, called *cyprine*—a Greek name for the "juice that flows from a woman making love"—diminish with age. Older family doctors may not know the problem exists, and we aren't particularly forthcoming in discussing it with younger doctors.

There are few satisfactory emollients to remedy the situation. I wrote to three pharmaceutical houses and a major cosmetics chain to draw their attention to the older woman's need for a suitable, easily applied, non-irritating vaginal lubricant. No luck. One company said it was not necessary to develop such a product, another said they are doing "all kinds of things to improve the lives of women, but this was not deemed in the best interests of the company," and the third said K-Y Jelly was adequate, and they were not interested. (Shades of cold speculums and rectal exams, not to mention the hospital smell!) Even a self-proclaimed sensitive and progressive cosmetics chain said they didn't see a need for such a product at this time. Dr. Marilyn Pratt, who recognized the need from her gynecological practice, developed an effective product called *Crème de la Femme.* She describes it as a fluid-film cream-jell. It is excellent, but difficult to find. There are others available, and not just in trendy condom stores or sex shops. AIDS Committee hotlines are well informed, and one can call them anonymously.

Even though established companies stand to make a profit from developing a product specifically for older women, their failure to recognize the need is another bit of evidence that Age Mates are not taken seriously.

One note of caution: Age Mates are as much at risk for sexually transmitted diseases, including HIV (the virus linked to AIDS), as any other sexually active person. You may find it embarrassing to talk about latex barriers with a lover—maybe for the first time ever!—but if he or she is fairly new in your life and one or both of you have had other partners, your health can depend on it. If you are both honest and loving, taking care of each other will deepen the intimacy.

Sexuality, as it changes over time, remains a factor in human relationships—in whatever way it finds expression. Among the most common characteristics of long sexual relationships are both shared and separate interests, and commitment to the partnership. The best marriages are fed by an enduring love and acceptance of one another. And sex is always in there someplace.

CHAPTER 15

LOOSE THREADS

A n inevitable byproduct of weaving life's tapestry is a pile of loose ends. Squiggly bits and pieces left over from old attitudes and habits creep in to confuse and confound our efforts to enjoy life. These tangled threads heap up like dustballs under the sideboard. Life, as with weaving, proceeds more smoothly after we tie off the loose ends. It's useful to examine them and clean them out, particularly since some of the worst began to accumulate in other time frames, long before we knew about the consequences and after we have forgotten the reasons we began.

KICKING BAD HABITS

We have to start with smoking. It was once so chic! Despite nausea and dizziness I taught myself to smoke at thirty-five because I was lonely, a stranger in a strange land, without friends or roots. Smoking was something to busy myself with on social occasions where everyone else knew each other. I could look at pictures on the wall and books in bookcases only so long before seeming rude, so I learned to smoke.

The worst of it is behind me now, but it provided many hours of solace. It was what I did through thick and thin for nearly forty years, and I miss it. Back then all manner of celebrities would "walk a mile for a Camel," and nine out of ten doctors preferred some brand I don't remember. Now everyone knows the bad things smoking does. The ailments to your lungs. Endangering others with sidestream smoke. Messy ash trays. The smell. Reduced lung capacity. So! It was a rotten way to deal with loneliness. The tobacco business made a fortune out of me. If I ever questioned the power of social change it is now, when the cigarette craving strikes!

Some medical studies say it is harder to quit smoking than to get off heroin! It surely is difficult, and nearly every substitute activity is either illegal, immoral or fattening as the saying goes. I chewed so much gum my jaws ached and sucked enough mints to pickle my tongue.

I wish someone would invent a ritual to take the place of smoking—the offering of small gifts, being thoughtful of one another, the moment of intimacy when someone lights your cigarette, a treat awarded for a job done, "I'll have a cigarette when I finish the dishes." A cigarette is a measure of time: "Let's have another before you go." Smoking is over-the-counter treatment for stress, a doing-something-for-myself routine. What a shame it does so many unkind things to a woman's body.

In a look-busy-at-all-costs society, smoking is a way to appear occupied. Sitting totally still is difficult for some of us, and it is hard to find anything worthwhile to do with one's hands. I go in for knitting in a big way. By now each friend and family member has several sweaters, an afghan or baby blanket, whatever I think they might use. The terrible thing is, I can knit and smoke too! Without a doubt my own best relief comes from playing solitaire. (Presently wearing out my third deck of cards.) Fiddling with playing cards isn't polite either, but it exercises the hands, occupies the mind in a superficial way, and permits that extra cup of after-dinner coffee without evoking a nicotine fit. What's really helpful are the times your partner will play a hand of gin rummy, poker, or whatever with you. All the better if the partner is trying to kick the habit too. It is a matter of substituting the "devil's pasteboards" for the "noxious weed." (What one can substitute for backsliding is still to be determined.) When backsliding happens, and it will, don't hate yourself. Just start again on the healthy, lonely, smokeless path.

But everyone *should* stop. Besides coating your lungs with tar, the residue of smoke, cigarettes are treated with so many chemicals to defeat disease-resistant pests that the chemicals may do as much harm to you and the environment as the soothing smoke, not to mention the bleaching agents used in the papers. Sometimes, when the craving gets terrible, your body may just be wanting a deep breath to swell out the lungs. Draw air in deeply as with inhaling, and blow it out slowly through the lips. It is even better if you can roll your tongue into a narrow tube. You may even be able to fool yourself!

The way I finally made the break was by selecting a prominent place for a large, hand-blown, Italian glass vase I had lugged home from a trip. Every day I *did not* buy a pack of cigarettes I put that amount of money into the vase. (Cigarettes then cost less than a fraction of what they cost now. My pension would *never* stand the strain today!) As I watched those bills pile up, I began to fantasize about all the great things I could do with the money. I even did some of them. Should have started much sooner. Had I put the money from thirty-nine years of smoking in that elegant vase, there would have been a Mercedes Benz parked out there instead of the faithful Honda. Next time backsliding rears its smoky head, I think I'll try "the patch." One friend tried it and within two months was smoke- and craving-free. She kept a little tube around to suck on for oral gratification. The main problem with the patch is that you must have a doctor's prescription and a lot of money to pay for them. Patches cost more than cigarettes, at least for the time being.

A similar devastating practice the flesh is heir to comes in a bottle, that magical genie that erases the moment's cares, eases some sorts of pain, and alters your mind. Alcohol—the oldest tranquilizer. It is a fine thing in moderation, but your needs may escalate beyond the point of pleasure into an addiction that ruins mental acuity, motor co-ordination, sleep, digestion and ultimately the whole person.

A before-dinner cocktail or glass of wine with meals is, generally speaking, a good thing—a digestive, a relaxant, and above all a pleasant social ritual. To refuse so gracious a custom is a shame, but to allow alcohol to take you to the point of addiction is all too often tragic.

With drinking, as with most things, we must know ourselves. There are no rules about quantity or how much alcohol is all right. The only barometer is the way an individual reacts. Some physiologies are more susceptible to the influence of alcohol than others, apparently because absorption rates differ or vary with body weight. For a few people, genetic makeup affects how much alcohol their systems can handle. Age alters the body's ability to tolerate alcohol, and the cumulative effect can build up almost without a person knowing what is happening.

Alcoholic dependence seriously limits your potential. If you sense that it is happening to you, get help. It is far too difficult and lonely to undertake self-treatment. There are support groups in nearly every community. If you tend to tie one on with a certain companion, cut the companion or just the drinking, whichever is easier. Sometimes vitamins help; ask your doctor. And don't drive. We need each other. All of us Age Mates need you! We have things to do together.

Write Down That Heavy Load

We carry so much mental stuff around with us—old tape loops, my partner calls them—ancient "should have done's," dozens of "I wish I'd said's," scathing put-downs that fester away for years, thwarted dreams, disappointments, abuse from long ago, sorrows, deprivations, and on and on and on, none of which you can do anything about now. Life is better if we can find a way to get rid of old injustices, grievances, hurts. We probably have a right to our indignation, but indignation doesn't hurt the bads; it just hurts us. Therefore let us consider this advice from a seven year-old:

> Writing is easy.
> I just sit down
> and write out my mind.

We all know the pen is mightier than the sword. Instead of slitting your throat (or someone else's), find an easy writing implement, some blank paper and a place to be alone, and become your own loving analyst. Next, set a time limit. Start with half an hour, and just write. Write anything that comes to mind, repeating yourself if necessary, although you never will. Don't worry about spelling and syntax, this is not for publication. If you are brooding about some rotten, sad or frightening event, write about that. If you are filled with loathing, write it out. You will be amazed at what happens.

Set topics for yourself. For example, I am unhappy because . . . I would feel better if . . . I am furious at my neighbor because . . .

That last topic had considerable relevance to my life. For most of a year, anger over my neighbor's ignorant selfishness spun riotously through my head every day as the cat and I walked up for the mail. I got furious just walking past the opening in the trees where I could see his house, more angry walking back. It spoiled the day, the walk and the pleasure of being in nature. That rich old man had acted crudely, blocking our road, clearcutting his forest, dumping stuff in our stream, and other anti-social doings. It filled me with rage and sent my cardiovascular rate into orbit. So one day I decided I would give the old fart a piece of my mind. I wrote five and a half pages in a fine fury, then stuffed them into a file folder until I could decide whether to mail them off or deliver them in person.

Well, guess what? Next day I noticed new leaves coming on the hawthorn and an interesting water plant sprouting near the outlet to the pond. The first of the little English daisies were blooming along the road. The breeze felt fresh and almost springlike. A bird scolded the cat. By the time I passed the neighbor's house I realized he hadn't even entered my mind. I didn't need to think about him because all his ugliness was stashed upstairs in a file folder, and still is. He's just as rotten as ever, but I'm not.

A number of counseling institutions suggest keeping a journal as a problem-solving or centering device. Adult education workshops in journal-keeping will help get you started. "Writing out" is constructive. It helps you see the problem from different points of view, experiment with different approaches. The act of writing is a way to order thoughts. Situations become clear with the simple act of setting them down word by word. Problems needing attention are illuminated somehow, and become more manageable.

Try it someday when you are really angry or unhappy. Write out your mind. Spare no metaphor! Let your ballpoint spew venom if the circumstances warrant. Since that neighborly incident, I've written out pages of annoyance and irritation—about mates, in-laws, kids, whatever. They are all stuffed in a file I don't even read, but the annoyances are pretty much gone. What is left of the angers can be looked at with far more objectivity. Writing out is a kind of mental laxative. You feel great when you finally move the – – it out!

These masterpieces are for you alone. Either keep them out of harm's way, or make a sacrificial offering to the Fire Goddess when their work is done. You will be surprised at how liberated you feel.

SAYING NO TO VIOLENCE

During these times of tattered morality the news contains disturbing accounts of abuse—abuse of children, inmates in correctional institutions and young boys in parochial schools. I wasn't aware of such things when my children were growing up, although I sensed terrible dis-ease when visiting the Indian Residential School in my town to prepare a television program on their work. The clues were there in the cheerless atmosphere and the somber expressions of the children. I failed to see what I was looking at and still hold myself responsible for not making it known to someone who could help.

We can see some of the same expressions in certain older people. Perhaps the cause can be found in reports of "elder abuse," disturbingly frequent in certain family situations and in institutions where the very old, incontinent and disabled are held. We might be able to help. Defenseless older people, usually women, are easy victims. Old people, four times as many women as men, are denied their selfhood, overmedicated, abused, cheated, isolated, physically attacked, robbed, and possibly assisted to premature death.

I've been unable to find information about elder abuse from earlier times, but undoubtedly it has existed in some degree throughout history. According to 1990 Canadian Department of Justice figures, 94 percent of personal assaults are perpetrated by men upon women. It happens in every part of society, not just among the poor and infirm. Some older women suffer abuse from their children or from care attendants. They may be "held up" for their pension checks, forced to sign over savings accounts, their homes or securities. For the good of us all this must not be tolerated!

Society's ready acceptance of violence is one of the byproducts of so many wars. In fact, Western tradition is a centuries-long story of violence, and women and children are often the victims. Remember the estimated millions of women burned alive in the name of religion between the thirteenth and the sixteenth centuries. Women were tied to trees and burned, tied to poles, drowned. Smothered sometimes. Hung quite often. Some of them were midwives and healers, practicing their arts as they had for centuries. They attended the dying and were condemned to death. They performed their traditional role helping women through childbirth and were condemned to death. It was a sin to ease the pain of birth. Although millions of the women killed were practicing Christians, the clergy condemned them as witches and ordered them burned alive. It was legal for the Church to claim the possessions of anyone accused of witchcraft. Their land, jewels, even their gowns became possessions of the Church. It is possible that you will see some of the valuables stolen from these millions in the bejeweled icons, altars and diadems of Europe. Eventually women were condemned for being old, for being knowledgeable or for having property and possessions the Church coveted. In some communities *all* women were exterminated. If you want to know more, I recommend "The Burning Times," a chapter in Starhawk's moving book, *Dreaming the Dark*.

It is painful to contemplate not only the suffering, but also the wisdom lost through these deaths, estimated to be half the women in Europe and England. Lost forever is their knowledge, their DNA, their experience and their creativity. These women—herbalists, healers caring for others—were turned to ashes without a trace, to extinguish the power of women. They were the scientists and doctors of the Dark Ages. They enjoyed prestige and respect in their communities. They knew and used herbs for treatments, could set bones, could treat and cleanse wounds with molds not unlike those in which penicillin was discovered centuries later. They prepared poultices and healing teas. They served suffering people with special knowledge and experience. Later, women helping women was deemed a crime against the church. Crones were executed because they demonstrated compassionate ways for human beings to relate to one another and acted to ease the lifelong misery favored by the priesthood. They were skilled in a fevered age when ignorance was in control, and they were women. That was enough. How can we hold any respect for a belief system so vulnerable to corruption and evil. We must remain on guard for any similar obscenities. Think for a moment of the parallels, as we hear rationalizations for continuing to build nuclear arsenals. Once the hatred was mainly for women; today it includes all humanity.

It is ironic that those four centuries of witch burning took place along with some of man's most civilized accomplishments. The depravity continued through the Protestant Reformation. The newly invented printing press spread the word of God. The Age of Exploration began with circumnavigation of the globe and the discovery of the New World, when a mere fifty years earlier Joan of Arc was burned alive. While Michelangelo and Leonardo painted the great masterpieces of the Renaissance, women were burned for their knowledge and healing powers while the Black Death raged unchecked. In Spain the Inquisition continued throughout the voyages of exploration and a blossoming of the arts. El Greco paints no smoke rising in his view over Toledo. Cervantes fought his literary injustices, but heard no cries of women dying from fire and torture.

The barbarism did not stop at Europe's shores. In colonial America, women were pilloried, drowned and burned at the stake at the urging of protestant preachers in the Massachusetts of the 1690s. Explorers carried the same institutions of power around the world. The "heathen" were robbed, enslaved, tortured and killed in colonies in the New World and all over the globe. Injustice scarcely rates historical mention.

Today, violence and the acceptance of violence gain momentum from the public's supposed preference for "hurt-and-kill" movies and television. Those who produce, sell and broadcast such material deliberately precipitate violence and underwrite its acceptability. Not infrequently, crimes bear more than passing resemblance to recent films or television episodes.

Violence for the sake of violence and explosive destruction of property prove we have so much, we can destroy anything we wish. It propagates ever more greedy consumption, and deteriorates into ever more acceptable "justice" dispensed from a gun.

Death is real, not casual entertainment. Exploitation of violent death is perpetrated by a society too squeamish to consider natural death in the order of things. We are told that this is what people want. It pays big at the box office. *Hurt-and-kill* has replaced the horse opera as Hollywood's major product, and it is exported all over the world. We are in serious need of a new definition of obscenity. If the present trend is carried to its logical conclusion, the entertainment industry will have blown up every structure and killed every human being on the planet. Then what will the tough guys do for amusement? We have voices and the right to protest.

This discussion is not intended as anti-men. I like men. "Some of my best friends are men." Nonetheless, cruelty is largely perpetrated by males in this and other societies. As proof that men are not the only ones responsible we are offered the "Bitch of Belsen" as an example of female cruelty. However evil she was, untold thousands of males carry out equally awful deeds and remain nameless. Women rarely make wars, torture, rape or ravage the countryside. But whatever the gender, it is the acceptance of *cruelty* that must be condemned.

Violence toward women is frequently forgiven by the courts, condoned by a system that loves to make the victim pay. "What did she do to provoke him?" "She had it coming to her." "She was just asking for it."

Being an older woman does not isolate us from the cruel and inhumane. That we are perceived as powerless makes our situation worse. An alarming number of Age Mates endure bodily and psychological abuse that borders on torture. Society, including the law, the medical profession and the clergy, is often unwilling to see the truth, or is simply incapable of dealing with it. Tyrants may develop more damaging behaviors as they age.

Retirement, or losing a job, can escalate or initiate battering. Bored, resentful husbands may let out their frustrations by verbally abusing and physically beating their wives. People in positions of power in whom we should be able to confide too often hold the typical belief that crimes of violence are perpetrated against young and attractive victims, or that battering and rape are sexually motivated. This is not the case, particularly with older women. Violence against women is an expression of power-over and contempt for the victim. Leah Cohen discusses these matters in depth, in her book *Small Expectations*. I strongly suggest you ask your library for it. It is an angry book, but there are conditions within our society that require anger. We must not be afraid to stand up for our rights, and shed the humiliation and embarrassment we feel. We are *not* helpless victims, but we need places of refuge. However sure we are that it will not happen to us, we will be well served if we know where help is available. It is difficult to find appropriate assistance when we are dealing with trauma. Many battered women, young and old, are physically unable to use the phone to get help. Ripping it out of the wall is a common batterer's trick.

Numerous studies in the past few years disclose that wife-battering cuts across class, race, education and income lines. It can happen to any of us. In addition to physical suffering, the humiliation is acute. Feelings of embarrassment, unworthiness and guilt play on the minds of all battered women, and are particularly difficult for Age Mates. Relatives and friends sometimes drift away from the battered woman, and the older wife feels particularly isolated. When the abuse goes on for a long time, self-image can be irrevocably damaged.

Rape of older women is also more common than we would like

to believe. Older rape victims are likely to suffer a decline in their physical health. The trauma of a rape can trigger a period of disturbing confusion and disorientation, requiring a longer period of therapy than for younger victims. As more and more cases come to light, we are learning that victims older than seventy tend to suffer internal injuries, abrasions and cuts. A significant number sustain such severe injuries that rape cases are beginning to be classified as attempted murder.

Violence against older women takes many forms, but the one we most fear is random physical violence on the streets. It is the most common concern of Age Mates I talk with in the United States. Several have horror stories to tell. The situation is made worse because poverty condemns many Age Mates to live in run-down, unsafe neighborhoods. Some older women are so paralyzed by fear that they cannot venture out alone. The US Department of Health, Education and Welfare reported in 1979 that older women perceived themselves as vulnerable because they knew that muggers, robbers, rapists and con artists stereotyped them as "physically weak, emotionally distressed, fearful, and incompetent."

Since this damning report, the fear of violence and crime has grown all over North America. It is devoutly to be hoped that this does not apply in your community. Male-dominated institutions have failed to condemn violence as unacceptable. Until there are fundamental changes in the values and ethics of our society, there seems little likelihood that we can expect much difference in the future. The only approach that may bring change for the better is action taken by women on their own behalf.

Efforts to secure protection for women are initiated almost entirely *by* women, as women begin to assert their right to a life without brutality. In a growing number of communities the campaign to "Take Back the Night" calls attention to women's determination to free themselves from the fear of city streets. Rape crisis hot-lines are quite widely available and there are branches of WAVAW—Women Against Violence Against Women—in many

Canadian communities. Shelters for battered women are increasing, but there are still far too few to meet the need. And shelters do not address the first question: What is wrong with a society that obliges women and children to leave the family home, live in unfamiliar circumstances and take the children away from school and friends, when the man is clearly the abuser? Why not lock him up, or pin him down somehow? This is a question men and their institutions must deal with. We have a responsibility to see that they do so.

In addition to becoming informed about the problem, is it not possible for women's organizations to select some part of it as their civic responsibility? Many of us are members of service clubs— business and professional women, university women, church groups, Eastern Star, Altrusa, Kinettes, legion auxiliaries, the American and Canadian Associations of Retired Persons (both of which are attempting to deal with the problem), and other groups, both local and national. Is it possible for an organization of which you are a member to take responsibility for setting up and/or funding a shelter, a group home, a haven for our older Age Mates? We already raise money for every conceivable kind of group and disease, support admirable facilities for children, care deeply about the needs of animals and sponsor a thousand other worthy causes. Might we also find opportunity to care for our own?

A Reminder for Caregivers

All that has been said about love and care for ailing partners, and much more, applies to those of us who are caring for aged parents. Ours has been called the "sandwich generation" for we are sometimes caring for our children *and* our parents. The states of fatigue reached by Age Mates in such situations is often truly daunting.

As you deal with these responsibilities, please remember that you are also in need of companionship, recreation and some personal happiness. Try not to permit guilt to overwhelm you. Value yourself and your needs as well as those to whom you are administering care. You will fill your responsibilities more ably if you avoid exhaustion. Take care of yourself. There are community agencies to advise and assist and enable you to take a break from longtime vigilance.

The main thing we "owe" our parents is to be the best possible humans we can be. That is why they raised us, and it is not possible for an exhausted, depressed woman, alone and without support, to achieve their expectations. Enlist the help of friends and community resources. And perhaps we could spell each other off.

THE TYRANT HUSBAND

There is a real-life version of the he-man whom many of us know too well. He is the Tyrant Husband. I know few Age Mates who have been beaten, but most have experienced the kind of abuse that undermines self-respect. It disparages our intelligence, and particularly our womanness.

The tyrant comes in many guises, beginning with the sort of husband who insists everything be done his way, for him, when he wants it. The demands include everything from how his wife packs his suitcase, to the meals she cooks, the way the kids are raised, sex, companions, and so on. He expects his domination to remain in effect forever despite any interests his wife might have. He may make his demands "nicely," but nevertheless expects her to anticipate his every need. Many, many unhappy Age Mates put up with this sort of tyranny because it is easier to do what he wants than to be assertive. Demands often increase as he ages.

For their lifetime together he expects her to jump at his command on pain of humiliation, ridicule and, too often, violence. He

240

keeps her dependent for money, denies her time with friends, continuously erodes her confidence, destroys her self-esteem and, last but not least, expects her to love him, care for him and laugh at his stupid jokes, often at her expense.

The tyrant husband doesn't change willingly. Why should he? Everything is just fine. The wife who gets brave enough to complain is ridiculed with a series of questions, such as: "What's the matter with you, anyway?" "What more do you want?" "If you are a real woman you will be content to be a wife and mother. That's what you are supposed to do." It's that last one that got me!

The worst part of it is these are the men we loved, the men we expected to share life's ups and downs and raise children with, support in sickness and in health. How many of us have been disillusioned in the course of many years is hard to say, but I've been greatly saddened to find too many intelligent, capable Age Mates forced to live as handmaidens to their husbands.

It is of course true that husbands who become ill require vigilant attention and often constant nursing. Too often he insists his wife, and only his wife, can care for him, sometimes on a twenty-four-hour basis. I have met exhausted women, selfless in their devotion to the point of being ill themselves. Often the husband fails to notice that his wife is drained and devitalized. He must be helped to understand that other qualified people can do some of the caregiving. Doctors could help a great deal by becoming more sensitive to the well-being of the primary caregiver, as well as the patient.

Because we love our ailing husbands, we will give them the time and attention they need. But we women have our own lives. Most of us will live many years longer than our partners. A widow in North America lives on an average of eighteen years without her spouse. We need to make some plans. Permitting ourselves to be enslaved makes it more difficult to pick up life's pieces when it is time to adjust to the widow's lifestyle. It may be unpleasant to think about these prospects, but that does not decrease the necessity of doing so.

I have seen timid, bedraggled women burst into flower within weeks of the funeral, free at last to live their own lives. It's tragic to wait so long.

The aged or seriously ill husband is not the only tyrant. Some men become tyrants on the wedding night, others mature into selfish dictators who use their wives as personal property. Such men are greatly to be pitied. It takes *so* much energy to be rotten all the time.

Retirement often requires massive readjustment, particularly for men who lived most of their lives at work. Many take out their insecurity on the closest person. That their frustrations are serious can be seen in the alarming percentage of men who die within the first year or two after quitting work. After a lifetime when work was his only identity, he has nothing left to do but die or terrorize his wife. Such men have always needed others to set the rules, to establish boundaries, time limits and schedules. Their own self-confidence is so low that they must have someone to dominate in order to define themselves. These men require counselling. By contrast, men in loving relationships live significantly longer.

You've probably heard the old joke, "I married him for better or worse, but not for lunch." I first heard it from the wife of a man who, upon retirement, lay down on the living room sofa with a stack of books. He was, he said, making up for all the time he didn't get a chance to read. For several months he arose only to renew the book supply, eat his meals or go to the bathroom. He rarely spoke and took no part in domestic tasks. In due course his wife, who had found rearing four children, cooking and housekeeping a chore for forty-five years, demanded to know when *she* would get to retire. He told her she didn't understand because she never had worked!

Finally she moved into a seniors' rest home, met some interesting women and men, and was very happy—until he moved in and renewed his exploitation. Then *she* died, her life still unlived.

There may not be a moral or conclusion to be drawn from this story, but I knew them both and it has haunted me for years. Her tyrant husband was a decent, intelligent man except for the way he treated his wife. He survived her by sixteen lonely years, still wondering why she had left him.

HOUSE RULES FOR HUSBANDS

As an encouragement to change longstanding behaviors and enjoy better health, longer life and more harmonious days and nights, a husband should repeat the following affirmations several times each day or whenever he finds himself slipping into the role of tyrant.

> I need not be helpless!
> I need not be lazy!
> I need not be boss.
> The women in my life have lives of their own.
> Their bodies belong to them, not to me.
> They are entitled to their own time
> and their own dreams.
> If they still love me,
> I am among the most fortunate of men.

Retirement and maturity are dramatic changes in everyone's life. They demand new ways of being. Re-evaluation of old habits and attitudes will be required of both partners. It probably will be more difficult for husbands to adjust to different hours, goals, expectations. But it can be wonderful—it's what most of us have dreamed of through the long years of work and responsibility. Like everything else of value, a good retirement cannot be purchased over the counter, not even with a credit card. We have to work for it. Some house rules may make for happier conjugal relations and longer, more harmonious maturity.

To Be a Perfect Retired Couple

1. Get your own second cup of coffee; you need the exercise.
2. Pick up your mess. Bending over is good for you.
3. Keep your act together. Mental deterioration is less rapid for active men and women. Exercise increases blood to the brain.
4. A marriage license is not a slave-owner's license.
5. Expect only reasonable demands for attention.
6. Say thank you, and don't nag.
7. Appreciate what others do for you.
8. Take time off, and vacations with pay. You're entitled.
9. Household labor is regulated under the UN's human rights code.
10. Men and women are equal in the sight of any reasonable government or god.
11. Your pension check is your own personal property.
12. Sexuality does not die out. Rekindle interest. Try a little tenderness.
13. You are each entitled to your own friends.
14. Respect each other's concerns and interests. Talk.
15. Get up and dance, and remember what brought you together.

Wholeness in any relationship can only proceed from equality, from the free will of free women and men. The loyalty of slave or indentured servant, while thought to be economical and supposedly trouble-free, proceeds from fear, not love.

Cherish your life's companion. Affectionate consideration nourishes men and women. It brings forth a flowering of personalities, enhances relationships. It creates that free-flowing, magnetically attractive energy which leads the seeker ever closer to the ageless dream of peace and love in the company of one another and God.

As Ken Keyes suggests in *Handbook to Higher Consciousness*, repeat over and over to yourself, "All ways Us living love."

NEW FAMILIES

The family, which we have always believed was the foundation of society, is being reinvented. The isolated nuclear family with father as boss is one of the shortest-lived family forms in history. It only came into being with the rise of industrialization. Due to greatly increased life expectancy the nuclear, power-over family is being transformed into forms more appropriate to the needs of an aging society.

Individual Age Mates will build the support groups in which we can help each other, while we are still able to make the contacts and develop the commitments to each other that will see us through the years ahead. Truly, old age is still a mystery, and forever a challenge. We can make it energetic, loving and power-ful—with each other's help.

If fate decrees that we live our last years without life's long companion, we will find in ourselves the strength and faith to create life situations anew. We have the model of earlier eras when aged women, because of their experience and memories, became a source of wisdom for those around them. They matured into the Elders, the Crones, the women of power. Society, and especially our daughters, need them as role models. To quote Leah Cohen again:

> I found that women who had a supportive and loving
> relationship with their grandmothers, aunts, or a family
> friend tended to be less obsessed with the negative aspects
> of aging. And if the older woman in their lives was a
> particularly powerful woman who was respected for her

intelligence, they were more likely to view life as a
continuum, with each stage offering interesting and
different possibilities. Old age became a natural part of the
life cycle and held out the promise of creativity and
fulfilment.   —*Small Expectations*

It is well for us to make friends among people of different ages, partly to avoid being the only one left among our friends, but more importantly to stimulate one another in a larger range of interests and activities. When we ourselves enter later age with strength and creativeness, we set an example for our younger friends and daughters. I am certain that we could be the last generation to be victimized by society's low opinion of age. We know who we are, and need not accept the narrow, ignorant definition foisted on us by those who fear their own aging.

THE RIGHT TO BE

These troublesome loose threads need attention if we are to improve the lives of women. The fault, dear friends, is not in our stars but in a society which rejects the value of women and the experience of age. Inhumanity toward women is part and parcel of patriarchy, built into our institutions.

We are in the midst of significant social change as we older women realize the possibility of pursuing our own goals. As we gain strength and confidence in each other the degrading attitudes toward us will change. Instead of passively accepting the old-fashioned notions that life is all but over, we can transform the last decades of our lives into a time of dynamic growth and maturity. Aging is an adventure.

We are the only ones who can stand up for our rights. It is up to us to insist on fairness from government, banks, housing authorities, family members and, especially, husbands. The only possible way to reverse the power imbalance is by taking control over our own lives, defining for ourselves our goals and our needs. It is not easy being an older woman in this culture. It is up to us to contest with groups or individuals who tell us how to act and expect our gratitude for meager handouts. We have a right to *be* on our own terms.

When the feminine qualities of nurture, conciliation and genuine care for others enter the mainstream of our cultural personality, we will be able to settle personal differences without violence toward the weak and helpless. A new and better way must be found—for the good of all. The world needs strong women in the council chambers of government, in the clergy and in the legal system. And do it in good humor.

Bedtime Story

You may celebrate diamonds and pearls,
let the luxury go to
your head
but nothing I got so improved my lot
as a thirty-nine inch single bed.
Once I thought that I was a twin
joined at the hip and the thigh
doomed to play spoon for the rest of my life
for that is the posture of every good wife
pressed in the mould till you die.
It was treason to ever advise that
sleeping alone was so prized
I dreamed of the day
when one just passed away.
Oh it's great when you haven't a brain

and your hormones declare you insane
but sooner or later you see
that a snore is a snore finally
and the breath on the back of your neck
is getting your nightgown all wet.
So you fire the first shot in a war
though you know there'll be blood on the
floor that will loose all your powers of
guilt and put sodden tears in your quilt.
For the role of dependence is reversed
In the sheets every rebel is cursed.
When the hand that you love
is heavy as lead, and you want to survive
get out of his bed.

—Gert Beadle

CHAPTER 16

WAYS AND MEANS

*"I live like a queen," she said, surveying her single
room with kitchenette, tiny bathroom, refrigerator and
television. "None of them had all these conveniences.
And I'm warm."* —Age Mate, 71

If there is one talent which distinguishes Age Mates it is the
ability to do more with less. Not one of more than two hundred
women I have talked with complained about money as such. It
remains a kind of taboo topic most would just as soon not discuss.
Women find ingenious ways of stretching their dollars. It becomes
a learning experience for thousands of women each year who find
themselves widowed, or alone with little or no money management
experience.

Statistics and broadcasters tell us that poor old women abound
but I don't know where they are. What I have seen are hundreds of
Age Mates carrying on their lives with competence, getting good
mileage out of their money. They buy carefully, dress comfortably
and appropriately. Even under greatly reduced circumstances,
Age Mates manage households, and cook and care for themselves
and their significant others with intelligence and imagination. Not

that there aren't problems, ups and downs, money shortages, even poverty, but my Age Mates have style! They rarely speak of themselves as "poor."

That is not to ignore the tragic needs of the truly indigent, the bag ladies, the homeless. They are real. They face arduous trials and immense difficulty, but their numbers are comparatively small, and their problems are not always economic in origin. When we see how well women sixty and older manage their financial lives, we can have confidence in our own abilities to make do. According to Statistics Canada, in 1990, 80 percent of elderly women lived on less than $10,000 a year, most of it coming from government pensions. Pensions come to women in their own names; the elderly, widows, wives of veterans, and so on.

Most elderly people in North America are quite pleased with their personal lives. (In contrast, only half the people between the ages of eighteen and forty-nine say they are very satisfied with their lives.) Surely we have something going for us besides money! We keep ourselves together with our skills, and we don't worry so much about keeping up appearances. Our pensions as single older women amount to a guaranteed annual wage and I, for one, think it is *wonderful!* It arrives regularly and relieves worry about when and where the next money is coming from. It permits me to maintain my independence, live my own life, and notice the days between now and when the next check will arrive. I cherish the freedom this gives me. I run my life on the *Laziness Principle*.

Simply stated, the Laziness Principle says, Do all you possibly can with the least possible effort and some style! It serves me well as I seek to simplify my life.

> Freedom is being free of what others think of me.
> —Age Mate, 68

Since society doesn't seem to notice me, I am free to follow my interests, exercise my curiosity, and try out new ideas. I can go where the gas in my Honda will take me and ride free rides on ferries between Monday and Thursday, statutory holidays excepted. Every day is technically a holiday if I choose to make it so. I can sleep as long as I wish in the morning, stay up as late as I wish at night, and sometimes luxuriate in an afternoon nap. At long last it is possible to follow *my* diurnal rhythm instead of measuring time by job requirements or when the school bus comes. Quality-of-life time has arrived. You tend to get out of life what you expect, so expect the best. You may already have it!

Most of us want a simpler, less encumbered lifestyle, and it is easier on the environment than the way we lived in our more fashionable days. We know what value means. We know how to shop economically, we understand about loss leaders, seasonal foods and Seniors' Days. Since we have accumulated an abundance of stuff, there is not much to tempt us into impulse buying as long as we stay out of the grandchildren's departments.

We've all heard the expression, "Money isn't everything, but it's far above second place." I am less sure of this as the years go by. Some very wealthy Age Mates are the most miserable. They don't know what to do! Actually there isn't much we *have* to do except make a commitment to life, not to possessions, position or status. When it seems, momentarily, as if life is over, seriously check out the possibilities. Inventory your own special situation. This you will recognize as counting your blessings. It is a different kind of financial statement, with values money cannot buy.

For myself, I'm alive. I'm healthy. My kids manage to live useful lives without emphasizing money as the first consideration. My beloved granddaughters are healthy and endlessly fascinating. The roof is sound. The well is half-full of water. The cat is fully recovered from her fight with the neighbor's tom. A few tomatoes ripen every day, and the wild blackberries are abundant this year. The compost pile is working efficiently. I can go to a doctor if I feel rotten. My car is holding up for its eighth year. The fridge works. Most of the money for taxes and insurance is accumulating in a savings account, and I have no debts. There is a good library in my community and several senior centers. I volunteer with environmental groups and feel in my heart that they and the Earth have need of my work. It is a very good year, give or take the political climate and the state of the planet. And this book, about which I care deeply, is nearly finished. I have enough!

It appears that money *doesn't* buy contentment—or maybe it does, but for whom? Ken Dychtwald, in his 1989 book *Age Wave*, presents a comprehensive picture of the financial power of North America's aging population. His point is that there are great opportunities for making money from us. We elders are one-fourth of the total North American population. He reports that these men and women own 77 percent of all financial assets and own 80 percent of all the money in savings and loan institutions. They purchase 43 percent of all new cars, and nearly half of all luxury cars, spend more money on travel and recreation than any other age group, and purchase 80 percent of all luxury travel. As a group these affluent elders spend more on health and personal care products, more per capita in the grocery store, and overall account for a whopping 40 percent of total consumer demand. Dychtwald makes no mention of what part of this money belongs to women and how much is under the control of men. Women are 67 percent of the over-fifty group. But for sure, he didn't interview me!

All this may only prove that there are, as some wag reported, "lies, damn lies, and statistics." It is clear that *how we use* our money is as important as *how much money we use.* If nothing else, it demonstrates the value of experience.

Money is that for which we exchange our life energy. It is a commodity, not a value. One can say that the life energy we spent as wives and mothers, culture-givers, and all the other work women do, is finally being exchanged for money—pension money. In this culture where women's work doesn't figure in the *gross* national product because we "don't really work," small pensions are considered our just reward. We should be aware of the discrepancy between males' and females' income, which is why initiatives like the Equal Rights Amendment are so important. We need to consider them for our daughters, if not for ourselves.

Lou Glasse, president of the Older Women's League (OWL) in Washington, DC, points out that most women over sixty-five were full-time housewives who worked at outside jobs sporadically, if at all. "Our Social Security benefits are lower than men's," she says, "and we have not generally been able to save the kind of money that would protect us from poverty during our older years."

In 1987, a US survey revealed that 28 percent of elderly people living alone have annual incomes *below* the magical sum of $5,100 then considered to be the poverty line in the US. Widows of war veterans are held to the same line, without transferable pensions or help with hearing devices, teeth, eyeglasses and so on. This proved very difficult for my mother during her eighteen years of widowhood, especially since she didn't want to tell us or ask for help. Canadian women are far better off due to the level of health care we enjoy. We need not fear a sick and penniless old age in the way our sisters in the States fear it. Older women also carry on the Biblical injunction that it is more blessed to give than to receive, sending money to the children four times as often as they assist us!!

Our genius for survival does not alter the fact that women are subject to financial discrimination. Of women sixty-five and older who are single, widowed, separated or divorced, two out of three suffer financial hardship. Among the hardest hit are divorcees. According to Leah Cohen (*Small Expectations*) and contrary to popular mythology about greedy women fleecing their husbands in divorce settlements, only 4 percent of divorced women in the US receive alimony.

Government and industry *officially* discriminate against women. We are paid less on the job, dismissed first, and receive a fraction of our husband's pensions as spousal allowances. Some industrial pensions do not recognize the wife at all. When her husband dies she is left without income, receiving nothing for the years of work she performed to make *him* into a responsible worker. The ills and injustice of these practices can best be fought on a grand scale. Individual efforts are worth undertaking, but too often left crying in the wind, given that the courts are deeply rooted in centuries of patriarchy. That's why there are organizations like the American Association of Retired Persons (AARP) and the equivalent Canadian group (with the unfortunate acronym CARP). Canada also has the National Action Committee on the Status of Women to speak for us. In the US, the Equal Rights Amendment (ERA) remains in limbo. These efforts deserve our awareness and support as both are scheduled for drastic budget cuts. We all know the unorganized get hit hardest, and the most vulnerable of all are elderly women and single women with children.

Women in the US have displayed political muscle under the name of Displaced Homemakers. (Laurie Shields and the late Tish Sommers were the two principal organizers.) Displaced Homemakers represents between 5 and 6 million American women.

Another women's political action group in the US is the Gray Panthers, organized in 1972 by the remarkable Maggie Kuhn. Panthers are dedicated to eradicating ageism by liberating older Americans from the "paternalism and oppression with which society keeps them powerless." They call for political activism in old age. I agree.

We are capable of organizing on our own behalf. Our power is the weight of our votes. We senior women would be well advised to make common cause with younger women. Fifteen million US women and 1.3 million Canadian women (our daughters) run the risk of becoming Displaced Homemakers in the next few years. The group in the United States has succeeded in crossing the usual boundaries of race, religion and political affiliation. Next obstacle is overcoming the boundary between young and old. We will need to make the overtures. Young women may not want to see us, but before long they will *be* us. Working together we should be able to head the oppressors off at the pass.

Power brokers and policy makers maintain an alarming number of myths about the ignorance of women, and they are not about to make special considerations for *older* women. We shall have to insist that they know how we feel about our situation. The greater number of women elected to Parliament and Congress offers possibilities we have not had before, but we must keep reminding them that we have millions of votes among us, votes which will grow in number when women born during the baby boom reach retirement. Our political clout grows with each passing year. Women are more than half the population, we vote, and we can run for political office. I know because I tried it—twice—and although I was far from "winning" either time, it was possible to inject issues into the campaign which other candidates had to consider.

It isn't enough just to manage heroically. Canadian women in particular need to organize to increase our political strength. We might try thinking about political action as aerobic exercise. Fury at the unfairness of women's treatment can set a cardio-vascular system on overdrive!

The philosophy of the bottom line prevents us from seeing real issues. The media and the opposition ask first, "How much does it cost?" when cost is clearly only one consideration. Where are values, quality, consequences? Women could teach politicians a much-needed lesson. With the wisdom of our years, we know to look for appropriateness, durability, serviceability, and whether or not a policy fits harmoniously into the whole.

Age Mates have seen the economic conditions of ordinary people come full circle—from the bread lines of the thirties to the food banks of the nineties. We sense it is a different kind of poverty that plagues us now. In the olden days we believed that if we were careful and worked hard, we could get out of poverty and into the promise of the American Dream, or the Canadian Dream. If we start out poor these days, we likely stay poor, since we are denied access to the education and skills with which to pull up the bootstraps. Unless, of course, "they" arrange for another shooting/bombing war like the one that cured the last Depression. Only this time, no one will "win."

For the elderly, what we have is likely what we will get, unless there is a major change. The law says that estranged husbands are supposed to divide private pensions with us, but we often require the court to enforce it. Thanks to government pension-indexing, small though it is, some of the rise in the cost of living is compensated for. Someday the rate of pension increase may match the increase in postage rates. It would be two-and-a-half times greater than at present.

Did you notice that when our pensions went up by about 3 percent, the papers announced that the president of some large bank received a 30 percent salary increase, or that your legislators voted themselves hefty raises to cover rising inflation? Then governments have the audacity to hint "they" may not be able to afford all us old folks much longer. It is time to heed the OWL slogan: *Organize: Don't Agonize!*

Our chances to acquire additional funds are slim. Few of us can expect to inherit wealth at this time of life, and employment opportunities for mature women are few.

I was fifty-five when I moved west, confident of finding employment. I had just stepped down as co-ordinator of a national foundation, and collected good fees as lecturer/consultant for schools and government agencies. I had been successful in women's terms. With a sudden change of government, our core funding vanished, and it seemed more desirable to be unemployed in Beautiful British Columbia than in cold, wintry Ottawa, so I moved west expecting to work in my field.

Not so! The first year was very scary. I managed food money most of the summer by collecting Sunday morning beer bottles thrown into the shrubbery near the college during Saturday night parties. Within the first two months I applied for twenty-two positions, each of which I was well-qualified to perform. No dice. There were polite explanations of why I would not be hired, overqualified being the reason most frequently given. Being female apparently was secondary. In all fairness to the equal rights legislation, my male partner got a similar response a few months later. In Canada there is limited opportunity for workers or professionals over fifty, and not much of a chance to find or keep any employment after the mandatory retirement age of sixty-five.

Retirement rules are more lenient in the States. Congress pushed the retirement age to seventy and then, in 1986, abolished it altogether largely due to pressure from organizations such as the American Association of Retired Persons. Although it was written into law, the reality was quite different. The workplace eased out its over-fifty workers, and hundreds of thousands of older Americans were either laid off or forced into retirement.

Few Age Mates can realistically expect to re-enter the paid workforce. The skills we acquired in our youth are long outdated. What good are five perfect carbon copies in the age of the photocopier? Word processors have taken over from typists. Fax machines, modems and dictaphones have replaced stenographers on the information highway. Teaching is quite a different profession than when we were recruited to teach at eighteen or nineteen after a year in "normal" school. In the fields of nursing and social work, longer training periods, new machines and new methods have eroded our employability. The attributes of caring, nurturing, instructing and safeguarding the young and elderly have been taken over by professionals jealously protective of their hard-won positions.

So what's a body to do? The only answers I have found for women not yet of pensionable age are to explore, experiment or invent their own employment. Three realities seem to determine the economic life of an individual or a society:

1. *Survival*—food, clothing and shelter, and a way to get around.

2. *Convenience*—things like telephones, recreation, television, private automobiles, and I would include books, music, plants and food for the cats.

3. *Illusions*—personal prestige, latest fashions, fancy cars, prestigious homes and monuments, and particularly those costly military myths derived from "great nation hangups," which the taxpayer is expected to purchase.

Let's begin with shelter. Women need homes, and nearly all of us wish to live in our own spaces. Whether a thatched hut, a single room or a castle, home is woman's base. That apparently has a lot to do with the way we grow old and why women age with more grace and dignity than do men. We know how to make a home out of almost any place. Eighty percent of older women in North America live alone; only 15 percent of men are able to do so.

Rent is the single largest expenditure for most of us, and this is where we are most vulnerable. Gouging is in. We should create special awards for landlords who are neither greedy nor stingy. Bake them some cookies every now and then, if you are fortunate enough to have a real landlord and not a corporate entity.

An awful thing happening in cities across North America is the demolition of affordable housing to make way for monster houses and high-priced condos. The coin we pay for this greed-driven assault is our sense of security and self-sufficiency, not to mention urban esthetics.

Women who own their homes often find it difficult to manage upkeep, mortgage payments, taxes, heat, and so on. Widows in particular may find themselves house-rich and cash-poor when deprived of their husband's income. Look into deferring property taxes until such time as the house is sold, either as part of the estate or when you move to other quarters. In some places it is possible to contract for a reverse mortgage in which you receive a lump sum every month, eventually to be charged against the value of the home when it is sold.

Short of inventing more considerate landholders, one solution might be inventing rent insurance. If there can be health, car, earthquake and liability insurance, surely there can be rent insurance. It wouldn't solve all the problems, but it would offer some protection from gouging.

Another answer is co-operative housing. It was amusing to live with a bunch of Age Mates in university. The "Golden Girls" on television have been doing it humorously for years! Adjustments would be necessary of course, but none so great they couldn't be worked out among friends. The value of living with supportive people is beyond measure. The circumstance nearly all of us fear is finding ourselves alone, unable to get help. Therefore, prudently, let us prepare more congenial living arrangements in close contact with others. Think co-ops, and talk over the possibilities with your friends.

Housing co-operatives have interesting possibilities. A number of older women might pool their pensions and rent or purchase a large house where each has a private room and share the kitchen, garden, bathrooms and the other amenities like a real home. They either divide up maintenance tasks or hire younger people to do for them. One group of Age Mates in the US purchased a whole city block!

A step beyond that is building entire towns or villages for seniors. These are beautiful, convenient, often elegant, but expensive. Another homing/housing possibility exists in taking over abandoned one-industry towns. They exist here and there, many of them with all the amenities. One such place in British Columbia had over a hundred boarded up company-built houses, a small shopping center, a hospital/clinic, and a theater in which to show movies, hear speakers and present plays performed by the residents' drama club. There was an overgrown golf course, now in good shape, and tennis courts, and spaces for small gardens. Last I heard the town was about two-thirds occupied, with over a hundred senior citizens living in comfortable homes bought for a quarter of the cost of similar houses in busy cities. I've heard that some younger people actually lied about their age to be admitted! That's not a bad idea, either. Mixed age groups are stimulating.

While it might be desirable to hire a town manager and grounds-keepers for communal housing experiments, retirees have most of the necessary skills to make such projects work. Information about abandoned towns should be available from the Bureau of Municipalities. If they don't know, they should be able to tell you where to look. Military bases, now closing as part of our peace dividend, could house hundreds, maybe thousands, of Age Mates. There are communities to resettle in every province, and most states. It won't be downtown Toronto, New York or Boston, but it could be like the towns and villages we remember from long ago. These adventures, as well as being affordable, are the ultimate in 3-R—recycling, reusing and reducing the drain on nonrenewable resources.

Australia invented another problem-solving idea. They build Granny Flats—small, movable, fully equipped homes with kitchen, bathroom, sleeping quarters and living space. The units are delivered by truck to a foundation in the family's backyard where land is available, hooked up with residential water, electricity, and sewage services, and presto—a home for an aging relative that is separate but near the family. The monthly rent is considerably less than a city apartment. When the home is no longer needed, it is picked up, refurbished and relocated. Here is another opportunity for entrepreneurs. The idea is spreading, and thousands of small, comfortable housing units would be welcome right across North America.

Researchers who study the housing needs of older people disagree on many things, except for two points. First, a variety of individual and group living arrangements are required to meet the interests, income and abilities of older people. And second, flexible arrangements are needed to allow people to stay in familiar settings as their needs change. Moving residence is stressful, and it can be extremely traumatic when we have to leave friends, churches and familiar surroundings. It is especially difficult when we "get moved" to places not of our own choosing. Think ahead, and check out various possibilities. You may find the place of your dreams.

The next greatest cost to Age Mates is usually food. We require less food to maintain health than in our more active life stages. Rich and costly foods are less in demand by elders as we tend to eat lower on the food chain. Hearing about the dangers of cholesterol, about half the women I have met no longer eat red meat. Not only is this a useful economy, but it is significantly important to the environment. In *Diet for a New America*, John Robbins estimates that it takes 20 pounds of grain and 130 gallons of water to produce one pound of red meat. When we eat the grain directly as good bread, cereals, muffins, tofu and so on, we improve our own nutrition and make less demand on the world's ability to feed her people.

The cost of medications is a problem for some. If you must take expensive drugs, get advice on where to find the best prices. Buy generic drugs wherever possible; they often cost less than half the price of brand-name drugs! The American Association for Retired People provides its members with medications and vitamins at good prices. Canada is about to introduce a similar plan. You will likely save the small membership fee on the first order of vitamins.

We probably have most of the furnishings and appliances we need. The silverware and dishes, pots and pans, and toasters so lovingly collected in our youth are now respectable antiques. That may be a blow to our egos, but it can be great for the wallet.

> Buy and experience,
> not a new couch!

Recreation costs less when you take advantage of senior discounts. Many of the recreational opportunities in your community are free or cost modest amounts for transportation and materials. If the activity you would like to try isn't offered at your center, community college or high school, request it, or hire someone to teach a group of Age Mates. You might consider teaching it yourself.

We are also ripe for travel. Travel agents should know the places and prices that will fit almost any interest. Check out Elderhostel in both Canada and the US. They offer everything from archeological digs to journeys in search of England's Arthurian legends, and much, much more. If we are ever going to travel and explore, this is the time.

Get what you want out of life. Decide what you wish to do, what you want to learn, where you would like to go. Where there is a goal there is a way to approach it, and the pursuit is often worth as much as the prize. If ready cash is unavailable and you have always wanted to cruise the Greek Islands, find out all you can about them. I know one woman who did just that. Then she signed on a cruise ship as an arts and crafts instructor. She worked four hours a day, enjoyed the people she met, and cruised for three glorious weeks. It is also possible to sign up as a volunteer for overseas service, making an opportunity not only to learn about but to be part of another culture, where your skills and experience are valued.

Cultural activities may occupy a bigger part of an Age Mate's life. Books, for example. Many that I didn't find time to read a few years ago are now available in secondhand book stores for a fraction of their original cost. Some stores accept your old books for trade or a small cash allowance. Take advantage of senior rates for plays and matinees, concerts and choral programs. Movie houses often have senior nights on first-run pictures, which are infinitely preferable to the popcorn-spattered mess on weekends.

Television is our chief form of entertainment. Use it thoughtfully. It is such a drag on mind and body to watch any old garbage. There are excellent programs that enlighten and delight, ones to anticipate with pleasure. Be sure to see those, but skip the hurt-

and-kill stuff and the inexhaustible laugh tracks. It is sort of spooky, but a broadcaster recently told me the people laughing on those tracks are long dead, taped during the 1950s when shows were funnier. Television is a remarkable, powerful medium with unlimited potential for enrichment and enjoyment. It is a crime against the creative process that it has been co-opted to hype junk, amplify decadence, and glorify violence among a seemingly endless parade of commercials. Television deserves better use. We are part of the audience and entitled to our opinions. Rumor has it that some stations, worried about declining audiences, welcome public reaction. Making your preferences known might encourage broadcasters to improve, maybe even include people like us in their programming. Some of us are "wired" into the Internet—the electronic highway which now blankets the world. The possibilities there are endless! Every topic one could wish to explore is there on some bulletin board or other. "Surfing the Internet" is positively hypnotic, but be warned about two things: a lot of it is garbage, and see that you don't become a mouse potato instead of a couch potato! We *could* make great use of the bulletin boards to organize!

Expenditures for clothes are necessary—for comfort and warmth, and to keep up the morale. But aren't great clothes hard to find? Our body changes don't fit the fashion industry's idea of clothes. (In my case the problem is sideways, Grandma.) Clever designers would find gold at the end of a rainbow of attractive Age Mate fashions. Women who know style, fabric and comfort can find a ready market in well-designed attractive clothing for the over-fifties. Because of our millions we are a great entrepreneurial opportunity!

I smile every time I pass the shop in my town with the name My Sister's Closet. Right! Wish I could have taken my sister Jean there. Better and better secondhand clothing is available. Some stores have ingenious marketing ideas and attractive displays. I get designer clothes at the GW Boutique, as a friend calls the Goodwill store. If you have never tried second-hand shopping, go with a friend and make an adventure out of it. Finally, since many of us remember how to sew, we might take it up again. Sewing gives us a world of interesting fabrics and colors, and custom fitting.

Good old-fashioned barter is another way to stretch finances. A Canadian invention, a nonprofit Local Employment Trading System, called LETS for short, ingeniously allows people to barter goods and services within a community. It is being widely applied in Australia where pioneers of the system say LETS improves local lifestyles, strengthens communities and takes some of the pain and boredom out of unemployment.

I visited Michael Linton, the inventor, in his home in Courtenay, BC, where one LETS participant was typing Michael's next press release in exchange for his help with heavy work in the garden. Barter certainly can stretch a pension and grows more significant with the layoff of skilled trades workers. You can "buy" almost anything with a combination of cash and LETS money—home repairs, massage, even housing—and build community spirit in the bargain.

This kind of exchange could make a huge difference in our lives, and go some distance in easing the strain on limited incomes. Some of the items of exchange which Age Mates supply are bookkeeping, art and music lessons, hand-knit sweaters, housesitting, babysitting, home-made jam, cookies and home baking, to name just a few. Information is available from most libraries. Find out if your community has such an exchange or look into starting one. You will meet some fascinating, self-actualizing people.

This chapter on managing money would not write itself until nearly the end. Since everyone's circumstances are different it was difficult to decide what to include. The reason I didn't want to face it is quite possibly because it really *must* include a section on making a will. What a gruesome thought, having to go through all your stuff, decide on who might want what, face up to all the things your life has acquired. If it is confession time now, I must admit that I have still to make a will, even though it has been on my "to do" list for over a decade. If procrastination can be elevated to an art form, it will happen for me around making a will. Reliable informants say you get a feeling of accomplishment and relief once it is done. I must do it! And so must you.

If you should depart this world without a will, the government gains significant benefits and your spouse and children get much less of your carefully gathered assets. A will, properly drawn up and legally witnessed, is an important deed to do for our survivors. No one likes to be reminded, but everyone—rich or poor—should plan for the inevitable to save hassles for those left behind. I suggest you consult an estate planner, who will often advise you for small fees, or for free in some cases. Once your assets are added up, you will likely be surprised at how much you are "worth" in the eyes of the law.

The first thing most people worry about in making a will is property—real estate or financial assets such as bank accounts, Retirement Savings Plans or insurance policies. You must name an executor, otherwise government agencies will take over at the expense of your survivors. The executor probably should be a person somewhat removed, rather than a close relative. It is difficult for a grieving person to make the necessary decisions wisely and impartially. Name your executor well beforehand.

Married people can designate each other as beneficiaries in jointly owned assets such as a home or bank accounts. In some jurisdictions this is done automatically, but check to be sure. I remember a young woman whose husband died in an automobile accident. All assets and their joint bank account were frozen. She was left without enough money in her own right to pay funeral expenses or feed her children. None of us need these problems at any age.

In the absence of a will, the law sets out minimum rules for distributing your assets. By naming a beneficiary, such as a spouse, we can avoid the process of probate. Probate is where the assets are frozen until the courts rule on the legitimacy of survivors. The process can take many months.

If beneficiaries are not named, all assets will be sold or liquidated, turned into a cash equivalent, and the money put into the estate where the tax collector takes his bite. For example, if you have accumulated $100,000 in home and accessories (given today's real estate prices, that is not so unusual) and just leave it to your "estate," your survivors can end up paying up to 50 percent tax. That leaves only $50,000 after tax—which won't buy much of a home for the survivor these days.

So do it, all of us! One can prepare a will with blank forms bought at a stationery store, fill it out and have it witnessed. For peace of mind, it is best to consult a lawyer. Estate planning can cost as little as $200 for a simple will.

Many Age Mates don't have a will, saying "Oh, I don't have anything worth mentioning," but everyone does. And get someone to photograph or videotape your special bequests so there will be no ambiguity about who gets your grandmother's silver vase or the stamp collection you started when you were eight.

As a final thought on wills, if your likely survivors are making it all right on their own, leave some of your assets to beneficiaries who will accomplish something with them. Every helping association, every arts and cultural organization, and every educational foundation needs funds. Your $500 makes a difference. If your life has been enriched through the arts, consider leaving some money to the National Endowment for the Arts, the Canada Council or a local arts group. Endow a scholarship or bursary for a bright student, give a dear friend a holiday of her heart's desire, send your grandchildren to camp, or leave them money for a microscope, a computer or an encyclopedia to discover the world around them. Your will is like a thoughtful Christmas list—one by which you will be remembered.

That's all I know about wills. There are numerous sources of information to assist us with this difficult, but necessary responsibility.

> One must honor one's unique predicament;
> one cannot imitate anther's.
> —*Bhagavad-Gita*

Our life experience has taught most of us to fear poverty, and for good reason. Poverty, along with loneliness and crime, is the fear mentioned most often by the elderly. The best way I have found to allay this anxiety is by adopting the philosophy of *voluntary simplicity*. Rather than attempt to turn back the clock or retrieve the past, we use our skills, ingenuity and compassion to move into the future constructively. Most of us have been through worse times. Remember the flour sack underwear, the agony of waiting for returning soldiers, the escapes from oppression, and the intense drama of childbearing. We are not really poor or underprivileged in world terms. Voluntary simplicity embraces both inner and outer dimensions of life and has its roots in ancient spiritual traditions and modern social change movements.

Conversations with Age Mates reveal that many of us have already chosen to live a simpler life and are being enriched by it. The concept includes the important affirmation to "live lightly on the land." The simple life, voluntarily chosen, is a way of living that promises enough for each of us, and with hope and wisdom, enough for many more of the world's people. It is emerging as a way in which individuals can choose to bring about a more realistic distribution of the world's resources.

An excellent book, *Voluntary Simplicity: An Ecological Lifestyle that Promotes Personal and Social Renewal*, by Duane Elgin, has just been reissued. Try to find it, for it reassures us of the values in deliberately, purposely choosing a life of simplicity. He urges us to be conscious of ourselves and and the actions we take throughout our lives. It is a kind of zen of living that promises serenity in contrast to the distracting bustle that often confounds our lives. It requires that we pay attention to our actions. Doing so becomes a kind of elegant game.

Living consciously fits with memory preservation and training. Thinking about what we do every day, and the effect this has on the greater picture, is both an exercise in self-preservation and a passport to contentment in a more harmonious world. Living consciously does not mean living in a primitive manner, but rather bringing the beauty of simplicity into our lives.

It affirms our ability to begin where we are. This philosophy is in the tradition of Gandhi, Thoreau and Jesus. It is the spirit of women who populated the frontier and created homes and communities in the wilderness. It is the lodestone of creativeness, a first step toward bringing both the material and the consciousness aspects of life in balance with each other. Elgin invites us to experience a more satisfying life.

Age Mates can understand this desire for simplicity, partly because we need to but also because we wish to. Maybe this is why there are so many of us—to set a pattern for future generations making use of all the skills, experience and ingenuity we have acquired in our long lifetimes.

We have lived through the most affluent era known in all of human history. Compared to any other time and place our generation has had *more*. Many of realize that it has not always brought happiness or contentment. We have time to try a better way, a simpler way. Voluntarily—before fate decrees less agreeable change.

100 Things to Do That Don't Cost Any Money

Preconditions: Turn Off the Television and . . .

1. Sit down and write your mind out
2. Phone a friend
3. Write a letter to cheer an elderly relative
4. Take a long drink of water
5. Pray for peace and understanding
6. Go for a walk
7. Do ten minutes of yoga
8. Give yourself a foot massage with hand lotion
9. Write down the last dream you remember
10. Wish for the best thing you can imagine
11. Compose a "when-I-was-little" story for a child
12. Mend the first thing you can find that needs mending
13. Write a note of appreciation
14. Go in search of your special tree
15. Visit the library
16. Select a book of interest
17. Read
18. Discuss what you've read with friends
19. Try a new recipe
20. Set your table with your best dishes, flowers, glassware, silver and greenery
21. Contemplate a lighted candle
22. Listen to music
23. Do a crossword puzzle
24. Cheer up someone who is ill
25. Make room in your home for a health-giving plant
26. Write a letter to the editor
27. Look through activity center bulletins
28. Go to an art gallery
29. Walk through some public place
30. Notice women wearing purple, and say hello!
31. See what people are carrying
32. Note the birds you see, listen for their song
33. Try to identify bird species
34. Take a "leaf" walk, noting the different kinds, shapes and colors of trees and shrubs
35. Brush your hair as many strokes as you are old
36. Sign up for a chorus or glee club
37. Tidy your closet
38. Phone Goodwill, Salvation Army, or someone who needs things
39. Check with your local volunteer bureau
40. Help someone
41. Wash your windows
42. Shine your silverware or polish the stainless steel
43. Learn another language
44. Dance
45. Do the colors, concentrate on how they make you feel
46. Look for wildflowers or for leaves turning colors
47. Inventory your skills
48. Decide on a new skill you would like to acquire
49. Imagine the world you want for your grandchildren
50. List what you can do to make it happen
51. Do exercises
52. Consult the Wise Woman who lives within
53. Write a poem describing sunrise
54. Breathe deeply to a count of four, hold for two, breathe out for six
55. Repeat five times today and every day
56. Give something away to someone who enjoys it
57. Study your face in the mirror and love it

58. Try a new hairdo
59. Compare the fragrances of your perfumes and colognes
60. Take canceled stamps off your old letters
61. Remember the events and places the stamps commemorate
62. Give them to a child or an organization that collects stamps for fundraising
63. Prepare to tell them the stories of the stamps
64. Look up the history of your community or neighborhood
65. Volunteer to conduct guided tours
66. Find out if your skills are needed by the Peace Corps or the Canadian International Development Agency
67. Choose a country that interests you, and learn about it
68. Write out your son/daughter's favorite recipes and send them copies for birthday presents
69. List all the popular songs you remember
70. Plan a potluck dinner
71. Dress up
72. Make up parodies of television commercials
73. Remember how to play the piano, knit, paint, etc.
74. Do a follow-up story on something you enjoyed
75. Read from a book of poetry
76. Try to walk about the house like Greta Garbo
77. Write out your grandmother's favorite sayings
78. Rearrange your furniture
79. Move pictures and calendars around
80. Check the dates on your pocket change
81. Take a long, warm, scented bath
82. Give yourself a pedicure
83. Read time on the back of your hand
84. Volunteer with your local environment group
85. Write to your Congressperson, your MLA, or MP
86. Make up informative commercials for the environment
87. Remember favorite foods with or without calories
88. Recall the taste of water in your childhood
89. List how electricity has changed your life
90. Separate your garbage and/or start a compost pile
91. Make two cloth grocery bags from scraps
92. Organize a car-pool outing
93. Return junk mail to the senders
94. Read John Robbins' *Diet for a New America*
95. Put a plastic bottle filled with sand or stones in the toilet tank to conserve water with each flush
96. Offer to help the school board with environmental studies, recycling, mending books . . .
97. Return recyclable bottles and cans
98. Meditate for twenty minutes
99. Visit your special tree
100. Look all about you and write out your heart

For invigorating renewal
Find a broom, a teddy bear, a pillow, or a friend . . .
and Dance!

CHAPTER 17

BRIDGING TROUBLED WATERS

O World, thou choosest not the better part!
It is not wisdom to be only wise,
And on the inward vision close the eyes,
But it is wisdom to believe the heart.
—George Santayana,
"O World, thou Choosest Not," 1894

What do we do when the heart is lonely? When we are depressed, hopeless, sad, embittered? Sometimes we feel unable to confront the emptiness, our feelings of worthlessness. Life seems pointless. There seem to be no recipes, injections or vitamin treatments to ease the hurt. Everyone feels the need for a bridge over troubled waters from time to time.

Shoving angst away is a wise thing to do when one is feeling strong, but when the whole world seems to be bearing down, it is not so easy to be wise. Merely to say the anxieties aren't real is dishonest. For the time being, they *are* real. They occupy our minds, encumber our bodies with pain and *dis*-ease, and cloud our days. But to sit there in the rain of discontent isn't wise either. We don't have time to endure depression for long. Better to look at each fearful ghost, acknowledge its existence, and hold up the proper charm to destroy its power.

One charm, of course, is humor. Betty Jardine did this for a group of writers attending a Women and Words retreat in Vancouver. She let us laugh at depression, age and body image, and gave me, at least, a hand up from the frustration of assorted immovable mental blocks. If it's not funny now, read it again and it will be.

Dear Louise . . .

I know it's been a long time since I last wrote, but I've been so depressed, I mean dee-pressed, Louise.

And don't tell me I'll get over it, Louise, because this you won't get over. I'm suddenly OLD, it's like I woke up one morning and there I was, OLD.

You know how the elastic in your underpants goes after too many washings? One minute they're hugging your waist and the next they are down around your ankles. Well, it was just like that. One day, my body seems to be hanging in there okay and the next, everything's sagging, like all those little elastics just bit the dust.

You know how I used to sneer at those women who went in for facelifts and tummy tucks? Well, God got me for that! I really understand them now because you really don't feel any different on the inside and then you look at the outside and you think, "There must be some mistake. I don't look like that." And you want to go out and get it fixed.

I should have spent more time lying down, I figure. That way gravity doesn't pull everything down. I had a girlfriend when I was in high school whose mother used to spend every afternoon flat on her back with lotion pads over her eyes. We'd go to her place after school and look in on her mother and I'd think "What's wrong with her?" Now I know nothing was wrong, she just understood gravity.

It's really affecting my life, Louise. Like last week, Richard, my son, the one that's going to UBC, asked me if I'd like to go for a swim and a sauna with him at the UBC pool. Seemed like a good idea. It was awful. There I am in the changing room with all these young things who look like teen-age boys, no hips, no bust, no lumps. There I am looking like Earth Mother. I try to psych myself into not being self-conscious. I speak to them in my head, "Look, you non-femmes, this is what a real woman looks like. We got breasts, we got hips, we got bellies." Anyway, nothing worked. I just got dressed again, went out and sat on a bench waiting for Richard.

What am I going to do, Louise! I can't go on like this for the rest of my life. I mean, I got at least twenty or thirty more years. I gotta find a way to feel okay about all this. You should be able to get points until you reach a perfect 10.

Checklist:

- ❏ Gray hair   1 point
- ❏ Baggy boobs   2 points
- ❏ Jelly arms   1 point
- ❏ Turkey neck   3 points . . .

Sometimes I wish I were an Indian woman. At least then I'd be called an elder and be respected. I guess that's the worst. You get to be invisible and nobody really listens to you any more or really looks at you.

Gee, Louise, I hope I'm not getting you down. You still look terrific, but then you're only 46. Signing off now. I'll write again, if I don't slash my wrists. Just kidding.

As ever,
Doris

Most of us have felt like writing such a letter. My own file would be six inches thick, and not as clever as Betty Jardine's. There's a temptation to call this "Feeling Sorry For Myself." But that's no fun. It is a rotten state of being, difficult to talk about, harder to define, and rather unpredictable. It is the seedbed of depression.

On the theory that things are easier to talk about if they have a name, I call this miserable feeling DBL. It won't be found in medical books, but then PMS (Pre-Menstrual Syndrome) wasn't there when we needed it. In my day PMS was when the kids got on your nerves, the house was a mess, your stomach ached, and the old man called to say he would be bringing his boss home to dinner after a game of golf. You felt holistically awful. There wasn't a handy excuse like PMS. How could there be? It didn't have a name. Which isn't the same as not having such a condition. Therefore, having not had the right to experience PMS when we needed to, in the interest of Age Mates everywhere, I am going to discuss DBL and what it does to you.

As mentioned in Chapter 13, the initials stand for *depression, boredom and loneliness*. We, and the medical profession, know about each one individually. Experience suggests that they cannot be separated realistically. The three states of unhappiness seem to seep together, reinforcing each other, spiraling downward.

The most studied of the three conditions is depression. It has been called the common cold of psychiatry and until fairly recently was frequently dismissed as another imagined ailment, particularly in older women. It was considered "normal" at our time of life.

Depression comes unbidden, often without a readily identifiable cause. Sometimes we can't even think of a reason for feeling down. Women seem to experience an increase in depression after the children leave home. No matter how honestly we wish them godspeed, the empty nest looms forlorn and unnaturally lonely. But there is far more to it than the loss of our mothering role. Sometimes we really don't know who *we* are after a life of love/service. We haven't had the leisure or the incentive to conduct a search of our own possibilities. This doesn't imply that possibilities are lacking. What is lacking is being able to talk about the hurt and emptiness and give it a name. We're told the mind and/or body always occupies itself with *something*! Nature apparently *cannot* endure a vacuum. DBL, anyone?

When depression hits, it is usually accompanied by a feeling of fragility, of worthlessness. Every bone and muscle calls for attention, refuses to notice the needs and existence of other bones and muscles. The body seems to work against itself, refusing the attentions of the logical mind. Even simple activities are too difficult. It is hard to get out of bed. Joints ache, back hurts, head drones, and on and on. Hypochondria, when even ordinary things seem ominous, feeds on itself and debilitates the whole body. (My story in Chapter 8, of discovering I had only ten years to live, is a classic case of DBL.)

It happens at some time to nearly everyone. It may appear just after a big task has been completed. A moment of exuberant rejoicing is all too often followed by a real downer. Talk to a mother a few days after her daughter's wedding. The bottom falls out of things. There's nothing to anticipate. Life seems to be coming apart. That's the empty nest, or empty desk. Many men also become depressed when they retire.

There are degrees of depression. The most severe type is still treated with electric shock in some institutions. As more and more physicians recognize the widespread needs of depressed patients, a growing assortment of medications and treatments are becoming available. Some are apparently promising alternatives to the mind-numbing antidepressants.

Please note that I am discussing only mild occurrences of depression. Persistent cases require medical treatment, and even hospitalization. Serious cases require specialized evaluation and may be part of what was once called manic/depressive disease, now called Mood Disorder Syndrome (MDS). According to recent reports, even serious MDS episodes are correctable in the majority of cases. Encouraging therapeutic developments are under way in several laboratories in Canada, the US and Europe.

The mild, recurring bouts of depression have an official name now, dyspimea—formerly known as "the blues." Baby blues, remember? It happens to about one in ten of us. We experience mood changes, energy falls off, we feel unworthy, inadequate, useless, and alone in the world. Sometimes even living seems pointless, which is why depression, boredom and loneliness fetch up together in my experience.

What to do about blues? It is debilitating. There is medication. Lots of medication, which seems to be the treatment of choice. But drugs mask the condition. They make us more compliant and manageable, but not necessarily better. Getting out of depression through what is called *cognitive therapy* is time-consuming for both patient and physician. It requires heavy mental work to look inside. Sometimes doctors are reluctant to begin long-term therapy with older patients. It is tempting and convenient to turn the depressed person into a passive pill popper.

Drugs aren't a long-term answer. It's too easy to develop a dependency, to get hooked needing ever larger doses. Mood-altering medicines twist your head around, can put you into vegetable land, and are extremely habit-forming. They are also expensive. Drugs affect individuals differently, and affect older persons in ways not always recognized by patient or physician. We are particularly susceptible to the hazards of overmedication and adverse drug reactions. It is useful to remember that three-hundred-year-old comment of Molière's that men die of their medicines, not their diseases. No doubt the same holds true for women. At any rate don't pill yourself, and don't let doctors pill you either. Don't permit them to medicalize unhappiness. We need to find better ways to treat life's troubles. Remembering how much great music has been born of the blues, maybe we can take hold of it and create our own songs on especially down days.

Vitality, not hilarity, is the opposite of depression.

DBL is the "blahs," the exact opposite of NAB (negativity, anger and bitterness), when all the juices are flowing in irritating swirls of destructive, stressful feelings. With NAB you want to stick around and fight it out. With DBL you don't care whether you live or die, and wouldn't know what to do if you did. After more than half a century of experiencing both depression and suicidal feelings, I have a cure, or at least a nonaddictive procedure that works. My prescription . . .

Recognize the ailment as a deception created by your mind. On the theory that it is darkest just before the dawn, and knowing DBL is likely temporary, sink into it. Be sure friends are within reach if it becomes too difficult to get out. Then begin to visualize light, the most magnificent, multicolored light you can imagine. Play with making it extraordinary. Shine it all around, wrap yourself in it, pour it over yourself. Create a cornucopia of light. Feel yourself becoming "enlightened" in the ordinary weigh, count and measure sense. The adventure begins now. . . .

The objective is to restore your vitality. Every living thing on the surface of Earth is affected by life-giving light. When you feel really down, when you feel it would be better to die, consciously think about this wonderful light until it becomes a vision. It will grow in your mind, becoming brighter, more profound, more magical, until gradually you will realize the depression is not so overwhelming and you are not so depressed after all. Boredom is illuminated by the light. It comforts me knowing that it is all right to be me. Sometimes imagining a sunny day works, but the rational mind says, "Don't try to fool me! Its gloomy outside." The light we seek to undo depression is internal, a gift from the healing mind.

Light is a wonder drug in the pharmacopoeia of the angels. Whether the light is real or not doesn't matter. If it relieves an unidentified ailment which has no proven safe medical management, it can do no harm to reach within one's own bag of miracles and reconstruct life in happiness and light. It cures in the same way a mother's kiss cured childhood traumas. Contemplation of the light possesses enough power to brighten the day and fend off the mysteries of the night.

The chief discovery is that the light is within me all the time and it is in you. It can be conjured up at will. It may take a day or two to work fully into one's awareness, but as the light grows and brightens, DBL diminishes and recedes. By the time it works its miracle, you will want to tell someone, talk to friends. You will find you are no longer seriously bored and the loneliness is ready to be cured.

Half of us experience depression or listlessness because physically we need more light. The problem is made worse by low levels of indoor lighting. Light levels in most homes are of an intensity of what is considered twilight outside. The confusion and disruption that sometimes overtakes elderly people at the end of the day has been given the name Sundowner's syndrome because of the changes sundown brings in the sensory environment.

It would make sense to turn the lights on earlier in the evening, possibly using bulbs of higher intensity. (Investigate the use of the new energy-efficient fluorescent bulbs.)

Other researchers have found that sitting in front of a light box containing full-spectrum fluorescent lights, for ten to fifteen minutes first thing in the morning, makes a difference in mood and outlook. Those of us who live in the northern parts of North America with fewer hours of daylight in winter are particularly subject to Sundowner's syndrome. You can make your own light box if you want to experiment with winter moods. Sweden, also a northern nation, has invented visors which shine two little lights on the forehead. Properly used, this invention is mood- correcting and energizing.

Depression is such a widespread source of unhappiness that scientists in laboratories around the world are seeking effective ways to deal with it. Much of their attention is centered on trying to understand more about the pineal gland, the tiny structure at the brain's center discussed in Chapter 8. It is known to be a light receptor in some species. Long a fascination to philosophers, mystics and biologists, the pineal gland apparently plays an important, but still undefined, part in controlling biological rhythms, including aging. It is known to be sensitive to both light and very weak electromagnetic fields. Through its production of melatonin, the pineal gland serves as a critical link between the brain and the immune system. It has been known for some time that immune systems decline as we age, but whether that is due to the passage of time or the slow accumulation of environmental influences, including radiation, is far from clear.

Remember how the kids condemned something they didn't like with a contemptuous "boooring!" Life is too short to permit boredom to take root. As described in *Positive Living and Health* by Mark Bricklin et al, our brains can turn into our worst enemy. The brain hates boredom so much that it will fasten on any straw to provide itself with some sort of challenge. The bored brain can so increase the dream capacity that weird and frightening dreams take over, causing physical restlessness or impulsive behavior, and may even inflict pain on the body in a last-ditch effort to provide itself with a new challenge.

Boredom is apparently the mental equivalent of the idle hands in the familiar adage, "the devil finds work for idle hands." There are things to learn and do out there, people to help, adventures to experience. If we wish to cure boredom, the first moves are up to us. Phone a friend, visit a recreation center, go to an art gallery, find a good book, follow your bliss. Look at the list of a hundred things to do that don't cost any money (Chapter 16). One of the more promising ways to reduce boredom is to exercise. Move around. Go outdoors, stretch, breathe deeply. Reconstruct in your mind's eye the sanctuary you visualized, and go there.

We each have a refuge which is always available, a place of discovery where boredom is unknown. It resides in the inner self, the source or the Life Force. It is that supply of infinite love, wisdom and energy in the universe. Once the tools become sophisticated enough and *real questions* are asked, that energy may eventually be understood as *life*. Every living thing holds within it a portion of life energy: some even call it God.

Call upon that Life Force. Talk to yourself. Affirm to yourself your value as a member of Earth's family. Tell yourself the things you would like to hear, and reinforce them until you believe in yourself. Say your affirmations. You are searching for your Higher Self. It may take some doing to arrange an introduction, but she is there for you. All the artists, composers, scientists, ambassadors, congresspeople, aristocrats, architects, statesmen, children, teachers, poets and peasants I've ever met have been a lot easier to contact than my own Higher Self. The difference was that I believed in them, but not always in myself.

All of us on a search for better ways to live have come across references to this Higher Self. We didn't always recognize her, but we experienced her often. It was that small, clear voice that told us to go to the baby's room just as she was about to fall from the crib, or the hunch that insisted we call unwilling boys inside just before a crazy driver skidded on the ice, scraped both curbs, and pivoted to a stop in the exact place where the game of shinny was in progress.

> Intuition is when you know something for sure without knowing it for certain.

Most of us have held ourselves open to the hunch, the gut feeling, the guess. It is part of our multisensory equipment, there to protect us and our families, and is often called "woman's intuition" with various inflections. We hear it in the "a woman always changes her mind" cliché. However much ridicule we endure, intuition is at least partly responsible for the survival of the human race, and will be an essential component in a better world.

From reading *many*, many books I have come to see these moments of insight and intuitive understanding as a manifestation

281

of the Higher Self. It is a power within us that allows us to see far, imagine how something might be, and create ways to cope with the possibilities or the limitations put upon us. So far, this intuitive knowing cannot be weighed, counted or measured, but neither can it be dismissed.

Kathleen Vande Kieft lists scores of striking accounts of intuition at work in her helpful book, *Innersource*:

> These experiences are evidence of a type of sense that is just as real as your sense of sight, sound, taste, smell, or touch. It is your sixth sense, your intuition. It is a message from your superconscious voice. Because it is an unseen dynamic, many people discount this sense, even when it speaks to them loudly. The mind usually protests this knowingness, for it (intuition) does not operate under the same constructs as logical thought. A loud ego will often drown out this small voice. It is easily covered, and not so easily uncovered. It is never, however, extinguished. Everyone has the potential of opening up to this unlimited channel within him- or herself. Whether or not you access this channel is simply a result of the clarity of your (mental) "plumbing."

Intuition is what gives you the uncanny knack for making the right choice among the opportunities that come your way in your personal and professional life. Intuition may be the best tool available to explore the unknown and discover its possibilities. Trust your own inner self to show you the problem in different lights. Intuition is a powerful asset in bridging troubled waters. When something goofs up, one can always say, "It seemed like a good idea at the time."

Listen carefully to your intuitive thoughts. They are extremely important to Age Mates who want to retain control over their own lives as we are poised here on the brink of the unknown.

Apprehension over what lies ahead is not to be mistaken for paranoia, but seen as the result of the culture's insistence that everyone fit some predetermined slot—for example, old is helpless, old is fearful, old is sexless. Old is often put in places where society can maintain power over it, measured by archaic assumptions. But we are truly different from the stereotype of age. Age Mates are vital, able, intelligent human beings with years of experience. We need not be victims!

When the only way to change is to venture into the unknown, when the facts are few or wrong, when there isn't time to gather more information, and when success depends on factors that have not yet materialized, that's the time to welcome intuition. Anything that can be imagined can be known. Intuition looks ahead, taps the imagination. It guides us on. Intuition has been called the mind's compass.

Loss of a life's companion, a child, a sister, or a special dream in which we found fulfillment and meaning for our lives; for all of these we grieve. Although it is a universal experience, I've found little in the literature to help us through such trauma. Ours is not a culture that allows raving and loud mourning to help dissipate the grief. Sometimes we barely tolerate tears.

Bereavement is most often a woman's special burden. As we live longer and longer we find ourselves increasingly alone, without the support of friends and loved ones who once provided life's framework. Now, perhaps more than at any other time, we need a safe way to cross the troubled waters.

For men as well as women the most difficult loss is the death of a life's companion. Nothing remains the same. The empty home festers with reminders. The widow hears his voice and answers, forgetting. She listens for his step on the porch, turns in bed expecting to find him there. She yearns for his touch, his arms around her. After a lifetime spent preparing his favorite dishes, she often eats improperly and can't think of anything that tastes good to her. She wonders where life's energy has gone, and why she was spared. Whether the loss be from death or desertion, all life's familiar patterns are disturbed.

Upon becoming a widow, Dr. Joyce Brothers learned that grief spares no one, not even an expert in psychology. In her book *Widowed,* she gives a moving account of the raw first year of widowhood. The first reaction she found was numbing shock, after which pain sets in. It may last from months to years, but must be endured before some kind of acceptance of the spouse's death is reached. Some of her advice to widows is:

> Don't be afraid to cry, tears are part of the healing.
> Avoid major decisions for at least a year. If that is not possible, get advice from professionals as well as relatives.
> Stay in charge of your life. Do not let others make decisions for you.
> Maintain a regular schedule.
> Plan ahead to avoid the trauma of anniversaries, holidays and weekends.
> Fight loneliness. Seek out new friends who did not know your husband.
> Get out of the house.
> Treat yourself.
> Exercise.
> Beware of pills and alcohol.
> Make specific plans for the future.
> Chart your progress.

For families and friends, Dr. Brothers advises:

> Write to the bereaved. Letters are very comforting.
> Avoid impossible questions such as "How are you?"
> Encourage a new widow to talk about her spouse. She needs to.

Let the widow cry. Do not assume her grief should be over
in a certain time period. Each grieves in her own way.
Stay in touch. Do not leave her to grieve on her own. Repeat
invitations until she is ready to accept them.
Refrain from giving advice.

There can be no doubt about the depth of the trauma. The effects
can be physically, mentally and psychologically damaging. Some
women, like Queen Victoria, carry grief to their graves. Sorrow
may turn to anger: "Why did he leave me like this?" "Did he die to
punish me?" Or more often, "What did I do wrong?" No one
understands the depth of grief, not even a widow's children. It is
an irrational time. "You live in a state of shock," says Hendrika van
Wouw, president of a ninety-member Widows' Association in
Victoria, BC. "There is anger, guilt, loneliness, disbelief. You
develop phobias; you're afraid that when you turn your back, your
house will burn down."

It will not seem so at the time of loss, but when the first sharp
grieving is past, instead of a downward spiral of despair, growth
will begin. Even at the funeral, one can celebrate the life of the
loved one, not the death. Look inside yourself for the light of a new
day, and accept the extra life you have been given. Many of us going
through the crisis of loss will find we are really ready to change.
Friends are of utmost importance at such times. With help, a
woman can take the opportunity to change even her self- image.
Self-image is learned and can be unlearned and relearned. Each of
us is important in and of herself.

Women who have experienced the loss of a husband asked me
to stress how important it is not to rush into anything in the throes
of deep grief, that it is unwise to make major changes in living
arrangements even when urged by adult children. The first year is
traumatic in the extreme and the temptation to fly off in every
direction must be resisted. Get sound financial advice; don't try to
make life decisions at the beginning. We need also to guard against

family members who arrive "to set things right" taking responsibility from the bereaved one in her uprooted condition. Despite their good intentions to care for her, she must prepare herself to take responsibility for her own life, think through her true desires, plan her life. Intuition will help if we allow ourselves to listen to that still small voice. Time and tears will eventually work their healing ways.

The women who are least vulnerable in their sorrows are those who have a number of friends nearby—the support groups I have mentioned frequently. Family networks—relations between sisters, and between brothers and sisters, often strengthen and give solace.

But there is another dimension, the one that holds the spirits of the dead close by, to guide and help us through the years. If the love relationship was strong, one's dreams may be filled with the loved one, with conversations, with advice, even with sexual love to the point of orgasm. These memories stem from our inner consciousness, easing the pain of grief. They never, I have been told, cause ill for the survivor, but are warm and gentle as they were in real life.

The grief most difficult to assuage is that which follows the death of a partner in an unhappy relationship. The sense of guilt is very hard to handle, and lasts a long time. The moral seems to be to get your relationships in order while it is still possible. Make peace with spouse, parents and children, for a loving relationship will go more softly into that bright night, replacing pain with the bitter-sweet memory of love.

Difficult as it is to accept death, other forms of grief may be almost equally debilitating. The worst, for many, is when a marriage breaks up and the woman feels abandoned, forsaken and desperately alone. One divorced woman in her late sixties said, "I would feel much differently as a widow. There is such difficulty dealing with rejection." No matter who leaves whom, mutual friends tend to vanish. Even when there is no fixing of fault there is a withdrawal of association. The partners have to find their own separate ways without their accustomed support. Friends once close to the couple disappear. A word of caution—don't oblige your children to take sides. They also feel the loss strongly, and may strike out, blaming one or the other parent. They will always need both parents. But that first Christmas alone can be terribly painful to anyone who has lost or left a partner, whatever the cause.

Some women move to a different community, finding it too difficult to attempt new relationships where they are well-known as part of a couple. No doubt it is every bit as difficult for a man, but he at least can begin his pursuit of women, an option not open to many women in a society where men of an eligible age are in short supply, where age differences are a taboo and where custom still discourages women from making the first move. Women over sixty outnumber men in a ratio about sixty to forty.

Grief cannot successfully be repressed or ignored; it demands one's attention. All one's intuition and self-respect will be called upon to make life whole again. If the marriage had been unhappy for some time, divorce only finalizes the drifting apart and, unlike death in a poor relationship, will be easier to handle. Nab the desire to fix blame or seek revenge. What's done is done. Look for new interests and get on with living. That's all that matters anyway. Be here now. We cannot change the past. Prepare to grow into new freedom.

We can also experience the classic symptoms of grief when a special project comes to ground, or a beloved pet dies. Days of tears may follow the loss of a job. The human person undergoes many traumas in a long life. Each loss can seem overwhelming. It takes much inner work to remember the deeper meaning amid these difficult experiences, namely that we have cared, we have loved, and we have been truly human.

We have a fantasy of permanence, that all things are forever. But nothing really is. Everything changes. Even the most constant of relationships, institutions, customs, habits—even the mountains change and seek new levels. All that is, or has been, was ours but for the moment. It lived in our souls, walked with us along the way, parted from us at the fork in the road, while we go on. Ever becoming.

For one brief hour
love held me by the hand
and in my soul came rising
insights, sure, profound.
I knew at once the nature of all things
as if some inner light shone through them
to illuminate their cause.

And I knew much more of me.
The chains that bound me
showed their cause,
and being found out, fell away
to leave me free—at peace
with one and all.
I learned of joy and laughter
born easy in the sparkling of a second
to rise in careless rapture to the skies.

But love has gone
it leaves me here, alone.
Still I am richer for its being
and in moments bare and dark
I call again the wonder of that light
thankful for the beauty
    of so rare a flight.

CHAPTER 18

GO SOFTLY INTO THAT BRIGHT LIGHT

We rarely speak about dying. A discussion of death is close to taboo. We entertain all things possible and impossible about life, but shield our candor when it is time to speak of life's last great revelation. Please do not be unnerved.

Each of us is haunted by fear of that ultimate Unknown, even as we know it awaits us. Whole books are written about aging without the word *death* even appearing in the index. With all our technology and sophistication, we, as generations before us, are afraid. Death-inspired thoughts and dreams unsettle us. We deny this universal experience even as we know it awaits us. Philosophers and poets have told us that all life is but a prelude to dying. Our moment will come as it comes to all living things.

Most of us would live more fully if we were able to cast off the terror by remembering that life cannot exist without death. Just as we cannot experience the majesty of mountains unless we see them from the valley, so it is with life and death. I have a true story to tell that may help release your fear. Although I devoutly hope it will not be too painful, I no longer fear my death. My trust comes from a tiny girl whose brief life long ago informed me of peace and comfort waiting at the end of earthly being. That comfort, strangely, is death itself.

Dying became very real one lovely spring day when the wild-flowers were in bloom. The experience remains vivid and is still suffused with wonder and awe after four decades. What took place along with the birth of my child is now called a Near Death Experience. In recent years, numerous such incidents have been reported, researched and documented—it is scarcely open to doubt these days. But at the time I was diagnosed as hysterical and threatened with incarceration in a mental ward. I was forbidden to discuss the experience. Electroshock was mentioned. Insanity was part of the diagnosis.

Back in the 1950s, the wisdom of science did not tolerate the Near Death Experience. However great my need to understand, there was no possibility to speak about it. Yet I never doubted the truth of the experience. It remains the most transcending event in my life. It is safe to tell the story now that I am old. I will relate it not for my sake, but for yours. It may bring you comfort when you most need it.

The experience began in an operating room of the University of Michigan teaching hospital in Ann Arbor. I was thirty-two years old, six and a half months pregnant and in the grip of enormous, fiery pain. Weeping. Weeping for the fate of my second, earnestly desired, female child. My first daughter had died four years earlier.

I lay on the table, cold and spreadeagled in their stirrups, exhausted from hours of labor. Tubes, wires, machines and many green-clad doctors and nurses surrounded me. Painful prods and pricks taunted my fading strength. My chest, sore from my beating heart, decided not to move for anything as trivial as breathing. A machine took over. Beyond the pain, all I felt was aching cold where transfusions entered both arms and my left ankle. The only warmth came from the spurts of blood between my knees. They diminished in strength with every heartbeat.

Somewhere behind me, a disembodied voice softly declared, "We're losing her." It was probably the unseen anesthetist who labored to keep the patient immobilized but conscious, lest he extinguish the small life trying to be born. The baby had no way through the thick placenta fastened over the cervix and up the presenting side of the uterus. This placement made a caesarean too risky for both of us. I heard my own weeping voice proclaim again and again, "Poor little girl. She won't live." I was suffused with sorrow.

Then, no longer tortured on that table, I found myself up above, looking down on the people concentrating intensely on some part of the shape that was me. They formed a little amphitheater of green-capped heads. Shiny gloved hands, engaged in some mysterious bloody rite, flashed in the strong light above the operating table. From my view near the ceiling I watched intently. After a while, I recognized the desperateness of their struggle and felt pity for them, pity for their earnest, futile efforts. I asked their forgiveness—and forgave them.

Liberated from the straps and tubes and needles, without pain, without a sense of body or blood, I saw the scene below transform, fade, and grow still. Warm darkness enfolded me. It was a blackness so profound I could feel its weight. It wrapped my cold body in velvety closeness. Nothing I ever imagined was more comforting than this deep, gentle, all-embracing blackness born of the void. I rested.

In some mysterious moment beyond time, I became aware of soft, radiant light. It grew in brightness. What intruder was this invading my luxurious blackness? I closed my eyes against it, feeling peaceful and well cared for in my dark cocoon, knowing no other need.

When I opened my eyes, the light grew, filling all the space around me. It was a warm light, as soft as springtime, clean as rain-washed sunrise, sweet as the clear, pure light of summer solstice. A translucent light, of a white so singular that all colors were visible within it—glowing, vibrating, being. This glorious light surrounding me, pulsed with beauty.

Deep, abiding peace flowed through me. I floated into wholeness and joy—free, happy, and at rest. Thankful as never before thankful, remembering nothing of pain or sorrow. Only being. There. Enfolded in Light.

I accepted this happy state, surrendered myself in it, comfortable and more content than any time in memory, until a thought, an idea, a voice (I know not which) spoke of two young boys. The unseen voice told me of their hopes, showed me their promise. I knew them well. They were my own sons, six and two years old—strong, full of life and needing only love and time. I felt my face smiling. My heart warmed with thoughts of them.

And so began a dialogue without words, a kind of thought exchange. Their father would tend them, my mind asserted. He could look after them, feed them. But would he? Would he find time enough and love enough to guide them, care for them? The silent dialogue continued. There must be love for beings so dear, my heart insisted. I remembered relatives—an aunt who would care for them, love them, and I thought it would be good because she was good. I remembered my childhood friend, Florence. Pretty Florence with every material privilege and opportunity but who was never only Florence. She was always the girl whose mother had died, whose father committed suicide, and who bears the burden to this day. There seemed to be no reasoned solution equal to the task before me.

I felt the love for my sons expand and become one with the Light, surrounding my thoughts of them with radiance. Somewhere beyond the Light my boys were entitled to a life as whole as love could make it, and of my own free will I chose to begin the journey back.

The Light retreated. It dimmed to reveal a circle of tense figures engaged with a lifeless shape. Stale blood odor seeped into my awareness. It was cold amid the clutter, noisy with the whir of machines. And voices.

"Wait! Maybe we're getting her back."

"Pulse faint."

"Is she shivering?!"

"Pulse still very faint. Bad color."

A louder, more authoritative voice took over, "This is close. Whole blood! A-positive!"

"No more thawed."

"Start plasma! *Stat!*"

"Please warm the plasma," I tried to shout as pain and bitter cold washed through me. The respirator filled and emptied. I was miserable to find myself again in that ugly place, angry that I had to return to the pain and heartache. I opened my eyes, but no one noticed. The oxygen mask severely limited my view. All I could see was a forest of transfusion stands surrounding the table, empty bottles, dangling tubes.

There was one other feature of the cold room. Beyond the doctors, next to the wall on the right was a blood-spattered instrument table. On it lay a still, crumpled bundle of hospital towels. It gave forth a tiny cry. "My baby," I tried to yell. I strained toward her with strapped down arms. I burst into uncontrollable weeping. Whatever I did resulted in a deep sweep of anesthetic, removing forever my link with the tiny wisp of life who told me of her victory with one faint, timid cry. Perhaps I was the only one who heard it.

I never saw her. Never held her in my arms. Never gave her my love or my breast. All parts of my women's body mourned—still mourn, remembering.

Two nights later she died; she, not I. And in my dream, in a fragment of that gentle Light, two strong woman's arms appeared holding a tiny body—a lovely infant, whole and healthy. Feet kicking, arms waving, and making the delightful small sounds happy babies make. A girl about as tall as a four-year-old materialized into the dream, silky red hair streaming down her back. She reached eagerly toward the baby. My heart surged full with joy as the older child cuddled the happy, bubbling infant. Her laughter sparkled. For a moment the Light waxed wondrously bright, then all the visions faded. I slept.

A nurse told me early the next morning they had been unable to save the baby, that she had not struggled, but slipped peacefully away. The bittersweet memory of the two small girls lives with me, especially in the springtime when the wildflowers bloom. I know they were together and well then, being in some other kind of life away from me, yet part of me. I rather expect to meet them somewhere in some other springtime.

Perhaps in the great cosmic order of things, a tiny girl endured her hazardous passage into our world to offer me a transcendent vision, to erase my age-old fear and leave me free. Could so short a life have been destined, through some karmic plan, to reveal Death—and Life—and Glory? Her gift comforts me every day of my life.

That experience still profoundly influences my life in many subtle ways. When fear comes upon me, an instantaneous glow of Light comes, vanishes, and lets me proceed. At the time, with all the medical propaganda saying it couldn't happen, I made an effort to reject the wonder of that Light. I truly feared they might put me in a mental institution because of it. Within recent years it is with gratitude that I have learned of similar experiences from others.

Even the hierarchies of medicine and religion recant sometimes. All these years later enough research has been done to establish that the Near Death Experience does in fact happen. Thousands of similar accounts have now been recorded. It occurs with remarkably similar characteristics in cultures around the globe.

Among those who study such things—anthropologists, mystics, psychiatrists, some physicians—the effect of an NDE is almost universally recognized as a transforming experience. Life is never quite the same again. The fear of death dissipates. Apparently there are no judges when death comes, despite the tales of terrible punishment with which we have been threatened all our lives. In that wondrous other plane of existence, everyone is accepted. The Near Death Experience has much to comfort us in our dangerous times.

This discovery renders the terrifying gatekeepers powerless, even harmful, in that they burden dying persons with doubts about their worthiness and deny them the mystery of Death. Many less rigid, less scientific cultures greet oncoming death with rituals of acceptance, escorting the dying person to the threshold of the journey. In such cultures Death comes as Spirit or Light, sometimes as a clown, not as a vengeful judge. The experience is told and retold in songs and legends, written into ancient scripture in languages of which we are today ignorant. Being human, we understand that we must die. Death, rebirth and renewal, the trinity described over and again by saints and seers, speaks of a beginning, not an end. Therefore, when the time comes, go gently into the peace and love and light which lie at the end of earthly existence. It is good.

In a 1975 book entitled *Life After Life,* Raymond Moody describes the remarkable mental journeys of people who have come close to death but have not died. These case histories are very like my own, undergoing the darkness, emerging into glorious Light. They are no longer taboo; there are now several hundred support groups to help people better understand these events. There is a scholarly journal and a newsletter published by Moody himself. While skeptics continue to find other causes, other researchers find more cases. The great universals discovered are that light and love await us in a kindly place, and that the returnees are profoundly changed by the experience.

Holger Kalweit is an ethnopsychologist with degrees in both psychology and cultural anthropology. He is the founder of the

Orpheus Project for the Study of Near Death Phenomena in Germany. In his 1984 book *Dreamtime and Inner Space*, Kalweit describes phenomena essentially the same as those I experienced in that Michigan operating room so long ago. After all that time, when I feared to break the taboo imposed by "professionals," it was with considerable relief that I read his work. Finally, after decades trying to suppress the memory of my own NDE, thanks to the researchers who believed the travelers' tales, I can finally admit the influence the experience has had in my own life. I wish for us all the freedom that results.

Predictably, conventional research has been busy with its tiny tools attempting to do the thing they do best—if it is not possible to weigh, count and measure transcendental events, then they can't possibly exist. NDEs are attributed to hallucinations, psychoactive drugs, traumatic experiences and excitation of the central nervous system, imitating a light effect. Others attribute it to diminished supply of oxygen to the posterior lobe of the brain where the visual cortex is located. But those of us who have been there know better, even though the NDE remains a mystery. After all, researchers, scientists and statisticians, for all their status and power, have failed, so far, to define *life*. Why should we expect them to define death? This task more clearly falls to philosophers, poets and lovers.

Every society from primitive times to the present has surrounded death with custom, ceremony, grave goods and ritual. Death holds such extraordinary fascination that lives of whole societies are lived in accordance with belief systems designed to assure members of the group that they (and often only they) will be taken into God's bosom when death comes.

Economies, power structures and whole systems of behavior are based on what customs and religions assume will usher the faithful into heaven. Woe be to the transgressor who finds it difficult to accept the precepts. Terrible tortures have been devised for, and far too often carried out on, persons who do not live according to rules made up by self-appointed gatekeepers.

My stern Baptist grandmother read me the entire book of Revelations before I got to third grade. It terrified me, tainted my dreams for many years, made me fearful and restricted my life. I still retain a shadow of that fear, wondering if something terrible is about to sweep down on me even as I write. Although the day is sunny, I'm half expecting a power failure, my computer rendered helpless on the edge of Armageddon. (Footnote: It *did* go off while I went up for the mail! So much for the worthlessness of superstition and the vigilance of our hydro crew.)

Among the few Age Mates who have been willing to discuss death and dying with me, it was clear that the topic comes to mind more often as the years add up. The emotional self is conditioned by the terror of godly punishment while the reasoning mind wants to find better ways of looking at death. The Spirit assures us that death is, after all, one more step in the nature of things.

Despite the great taboo around the topic, death is discussed rather more comfortably in relation to third persons, far away people—or in statistics. I don't think this helps very much, nor is it honest. I will die. We will die. Presidents and generals will die. When things get unbearably difficult or painful, I should have the *right* to die. Society and religion forbid death by suicide. In Canada and the US, some people—both patients and doctors—are challenging the law and legislators about life-and-death decisions. The conventional wisdom insists that one's life is supposed to be under the control of someone other than the self.

Public pressure is growing to draw up legislation which will permit an individual to make his or her own life-and-death decisions. The issue began to receive intense public scrutiny in June 1990 when a doctor in Michigan assisted a fifty-four-year-old woman, suffering from an incurable disease, to end her own life by releasing lethal chemicals provided by the doctor. There have been other, more recent cases, including the heroic efforts of the late Sue Rodriguez who took her fight to the highest courts in Canada. The laws here carry a fourteen-year penalty for anyone who counsels or assists a person to commit suicide, and are similarly severe in most American states, although it is still quite legal in many areas for the state to administer death through execution.

The movement for an international planned death policy includes efforts to gain legal acceptance of the living will, in which an individual can specify what procedure to follow in case of impending death, including organ donations, the right to refuse heroic medical intervention, and so on. Presently legal in thirty-two US states and before the legislature in others, the living will is an option available to many of us. The right to arrange one's own death is under study by the Hemlock Society, which takes its name from Socrates' death. These movements are growing at this time because of the increasing use of machines which prolong life artificially, even after vital functions have shut down and the patient is in coma.

Extreme confusion results from our culture's inability to accept the naturalness of death. Scientists and doctors develop ever more sophisticated technologies and interventions to cheat death, no matter how hopeless and miserable the patient. Death seems to be some sort of insult to all-powerful medical deities, and as our society grows more litigious, they become more reluctant to let nature take her course. Their miracles are welcomed when their clients wish to live, but there can be much pain all around when existence is prolonged artificially. Persons who have made peace with this life should have the right to let go.

Among other considerations, the horrific cost of valorous medicine must be looked at, particularly since it tends to ignore quality of life in favor of quantity only. An intensified search for more ethical attitudes arises at this particular time because of the increase in presently incurable diseases such as cancer, AIDS and Alzheimer's.

Until the individual's power over his or her own life is defined in law, it remains unacceptably complicated to plan for death in a dignified, loving way. To meet this situation the Hospice movement, begun some thirty years ago in England, is now nearly worldwide. It is staffed by volunteers in every community where it operates. The woman hospice worker I talked to was a kind of ministering angel. Hospice provides a place for the terminally ill to die with dignity among friends in the comfort of pleasant surroundings. Anyone can apply to spend their last days in Hospice, knowing that they will not be subjected to heroic medical intervention but allowed to die in peace. Admission to Hospice is open to anyone, and some facilities provide spaces for families to be near loved ones during their last days. Hospice is a profoundly humane organization.

We deserve legal permission for our wishes to be carried out. The legislation needs to be strong enough so it cannot be overruled by well-meaning families and/or zealous medical personnel. It is time the establishment relinquishes its burdensome control over dying. Certainly it does not hesitate to legitimize death by the state, by war, or by getting caught in crossfire. It's not morbid to decide how *you* wish your dying to proceed, just as it is not too soon to make out a will to distribute material possessions. What is most needed is a restructuring of the myths we live by, permitting faith and hope and love to re-enter our materialistic twentieth-century lives.

Fear of death reinforces the whole spectrum of ecclesiastical control, as churches promise believers life after death, *if* they spend a lifetime doing what the faith decrees and are finally judged acceptable by self-appointed human hierarchy. Our life conduct is conditioned by this obsession with death. It preys heavily on the minds of the elderly, as Simone de Beauvoir pointed out in her 1970 book *The Coming of Age.* How wonderful it would be, particularly for the very old, if we were to know a God of Love who would, without recriminations, accept us into all-inclusive love and peace and Light. Should not everyone's god wish to accept our departed spirits openly, generously, in the same way our Earth Mother provides for us throughout life, and receives our bodies back at death?

I shall plan my death and, I hope, the time. When goodbyes are said, happy memories recalled, a parting loving cup shared with a few close friends, I intend to die naturally at home. I have no wish for tubes and monitors, high-tech invasions, or heroic measures to turn dying into a failure of instruments rather than the passing of a Spirit. As one Age Mate told me, "I want to live until I die." We must insist on this privilege.

Once upon a time, when life was lived according to natural cycles, there were persons available to care for and comfort the terminally ill. They counseled the family, showed respect for their fears, surrounded the natural process with love and dignity. By tradition, the oldest, wisest women of the village were responsible for assisting the dying, comforting them, watching with them and, in spirit form, leading the way on the mysterious journey ahead. The wise old women prepared the body, conducted the funeral rites and, with ceremony, returned the remains to Mother Earth. We still acknowledge our antiquity with the ritual benediction, "Ashes to ashes, dust to dust."

The Death Crone, as the wise old woman was called, has all but disappeared from modern life. Except for the rare example of Mother Teresa, who eases the last hours of the poor and abandoned, and the work of Elisabeth Kübler-Ross, the dying rarely know a woman's hands. Death has been turned over to professionals, legalized, taken from the family and, most definitely, removed from the power of the dying person. It is now big business to die: the grieving family is urged to purchase expensive grave goods in the form of satin-lined caskets, embalming, cosmetic make-up, grave markers, and so on.

We need the Crone who once administered comfort where and when it was called for. Despite the scorn heaped on the Crone, I believe many elderly women retain in their collective memory something of the role women once played in ordering the cycles of life in the community.

We were the wise women. Our long memories prepared us to intervene with the powers of nature to pronounce oracles, advise about crops, preserve seeds, dispense wisdom and counsel harmonious relations within the group.

As midwives we were in attendance when life came into the world; we were there at the end of life to guide each Spirit home. We—Wise Woman, Crone, Elder—were the last souls seen by the departing Spirit. It was an honor to fill such a role. With gentleness and love the Crone made ready the dead and wrapped them in spices and grave clothes. She was there to assure a good death, as painless as her knowledge of herbs and medicines would permit.

There was comfort in this knowledge. I would like to think she will be waiting, wise and considerate, to ease my final hours. As it is, there is no way of knowing what strangers will attend my dying.

Among the ancient traditions of the Pacific coast is the belief that when the dying was done, the Crone carried the "bag of bones and skin," as the corpse was called, to the place where the Great Mother could receive it, freeing the Spirit to return to her star. The Crone occupied the place between the living and the dead. She completed the cycle, created the circumstances for regeneration. The Great Mother entrusted her elderly women with the holy duty to assure Nature's continuity.

> It was better for the world when the Crone was recognized
> as the embodiment of women's care for the dying and the
> dead. Women not only faced their own aging with pride
> rather than with shame; they also received due credit as
> priestesses of the final rites of passage, for their tenderness
> toward the terminally ill, and for the sacred duties that
> included their hands-on care.—Barbara G. Walker, *The Crone*

Much has changed since death passed from the hands of women.

In our age of consumerism, professionals inter the dead, manipulate and medicate the corpse, paint away the well-earned lines, return cosmetic blushes to the cheek and shroud the body not in love, but in consumer goods. These customs are among the most wasteful practices in this society. Our culture, brainwashed to fear death, pays high prices to remove the phenomenon from sight.

While funeral rites become more impersonal, and more lucrative, death itself gets further from reality. The changes are reflected in our language. We have a collective inability to speak of death. No one *dies* any more. They pass away, they are taken, they are called. As the whole event is removed from the life cycle, it is possible to distort it until it becomes trashy entertainment, a mere condiment added to thrillers on television, screen and radio.

Death sells. What *would* the entertainment industry do without gunfire, explosions, stabbings and torture among our amusements? Movies and television might improve if theatrical death weren't considered so entertaining. Death as entertainment becomes a temporary condition as the "dead" absurdly rise from television's morgue to appear in subsequent programs. In other times and places, entertainment value has been variously derived from bullfights, public executions, the deaths of gladiators—and even burning women at the stake.

Stern ecclesiastical gatekeepers won't let women pass unless we have lived in a manner acceptable to *them*. They crack lifelong whips across the tender portions of our lives to be sure that we conform. The punishments they pruriently imagined to keep us on the path they designed can only be seen as psychotic. Why would anyone of sane mind insist that "sinful" women burn in hell for behavior transgressions, most often having to do with male sexuality?

In the Crone's version the Spirit is free to seek its bliss. The body, tired and worn, returns to Earth. We will be less fearful when we allow Death itself to liberate the Spirit, allow it to fly free, as centuries of mystics affirm. Life is not an evil to be judged, restrained and punished, nor is Death.

Attitudes may be starting to change, thanks to wider contacts with world ideas and contemporary pioneers like Elisabeth Kübler-Ross. It is worth noting that just as we are returning to more holistic treatment of the dying, so are we permitting birth to occur in more loving circumstances with the aid of wise women.

Most written history has been about men killing. Unlimited funds, brilliant scientific minds and Earth's resources go to create machines of death. And men are *proud!* "Father" of the hydrogen bomb! Invention of nerve gas, of dynamite, even the simple little Gatling gun, are listed among men's great achievements. Let us oppose this insanity at every turn. Let us take death back as our sacred duty, and treat it kindly, with respect. The blood women shed is blood born from life. Man-shed war blood is obscene.

Think how we are brainwashed to support and venerate the powerful in their death rituals. Death is honored by millions of white crosses. Memorial Day poppies. Gold Star mothers of dead sons. Awards for conniving death, glory for military campaigns, honors for pointless slaughters, for serial wars never won, for inventing ever more efficient killing machines, deploying ever more deadly weapons, destroying bridges, water supplies, roads and harbors. Or the madness of the maddest—Mutual Assured Destruction—MAD for short. Crusades and holy wars, wars of all the ages, ancient and modern, serve war gods whose only appeasement is man-made death. By some irrational logic this kind of death is deemed worthy, honorable. We are supposed to tie a yellow ribbon around heroic bloodstains on the landscape.

The war to end all wars is on the drawing boards and no one is excluded. Should the decency and wisdom of humanity fail to prevent such a catastrophe, we will have to handle it ourselves. As with the hundreds of bodies bulldozed into Rwandan trenches, we know there are not enough priests, rabbis, preachers, shamans, mullahs or medicine men on the planet to pray all of us into any version of heaven or hell, no matter what bribe we offer.

For greater understanding of what it has meant historically to be female, I refer you to Starhawk, *Dreaming the Dark*; Barbara G. Walker, *The Crone*; Margo Adler, *Drawing Down the Moon*; Sonia Johnson, *Going Out of Our Minds*. Read *The Chalice and the Blade*, by Riane Eisler, for just a hint of the history coming to light now that women are speaking out against the forces that have brought the world to the edge of annihilation, and the planet herself to the brink of death. We must cherish woman's healing power as our legacy from women of the past.

However we may feel under siege as Age Mates, it is clear that we must join our sisters and do what we are able to do to grasp every prospect for sanity in an insane time. We need not question our qualifications nor the quality of the changes we can bring about. We do not have to make mistakes as awful as the mistakes made during centuries of patriarchy.

We can begin to reclaim death as our own, knowing it is a natural event, an interval past fear and close to loving. Let death come on wings of Light. Step through the veil of mystery unafraid. Don't let them drag your spirit, drugged and unconscious, into the unknown. Experience fully the miracle of the Light. My most fervent wish for my own dying is that it may come when my days are done, not when despots thrust it on me.

CHAPTER 19

FOLLOW YOUR BLISS

I like the sound of flags in scented wind
And haunting music written long ago.
And foreign lands and satin sands,
and snow.

I need the strength of trees and home,
The secret soul, the hidden flame subdued,
The comfort found in wooded lots, the
inner thoughts and solitude.

I love the mystery of stars and clouds,
And books with life and truth in every crease.
The music of the wind, and love
and peace.

— Alice Enid Schultz, age 15

The young poet didn't give these lovely thoughts a name, but her words come close to describing the qualities of happiness which most women value. This state of being, this fullness of spirit felt in some inner place, is wished for, dreamed of, envied and imagined. We have written the yearning for happiness into music and literature. It is enshrined but not defined in the US Declaration of Independence and the Canadian Bill of Rights. Happiness is nowhere and everywhere. It may be experienced during moments of solitude, at dinner, on a walk, in a song, the touch of a lover's lips, a glimpse of beauty, the exhilaration of a task well done, or when a tiny, trusting hand slips into yours. Happiness, mysterious and undefinable, is the most subjective of all our emotions.

Included in the rich heritage left to us by Joseph Campbell was his passionate discernment of the myths that guide our lives. He spoke of the need for new myths that would help us be more gentle to the Earth and to each other. A basic tenet was his idea of bliss. "What is happiness and how can we find it?" he was asked in many ways. His answer, unwavering, was simply: "Follow your bliss."

Not knowing what "bliss" actually is, I've puzzled over the meaning of Joseph Campbell's advice. I believed with all my North American, middle class, academic heart that the way to find out about something is to dissect and define what I wished to understand, seeking in ever greater depth what I wanted to know. No matter how far I traveled or how determined the effort, I came up short. I would return from my explorations with useful information, memorable experiences, enlightening observations, helpful insights, but never with happiness, let alone bliss. Sometimes it seemed as if I had gotten close to understanding, only to feel the fairy wisp of knowing flit beyond reach, beyond sight. Like everyone else, I've always wanted to be happy, but achieved the feeling only rarely, fleetingly, and nearly always in the presence of nature's miracles.

Now I think I know where bliss comes from. It comes from the way your soul looks at where you are. The story of a young mother in Salt Lake City stays with me. She lived in a cheerless basement apartment. Her toddler was one of those hyper, healthy little creatures, into everything. She worked twelve-hour shifts as a night nurse, and then she had a week off duty. She sang or whistled as she washed and cleaned and played with the child. A few days later, very tired after a long shift, she told me that her week off was the happiest time she could remember.

Her bliss surely came from her life force deep inside, for hers was far from an easy life, lacking possessions, even opportunity. She accepted her situation, her self and her loved ones. She had found happiness where many of us would find drudgery. Where there is acceptance of the self, where character and personality are not compared, where flaws of body, mind and manner are not judged is, perhaps, the place where happiness lives, where one can say, "I am content."

That's what my son told me decades ago: "Look inside, Mom. You'll find everything you need to know." His suggestion seemed improbable, much too painful, and a little ridiculous. It was too simple. Advice from a teenager, after all! The truth is that I was afraid to look inside. I stopped short of scoffing at his advice, but felt helpless before it. I was afraid of what I would find, or what I wouldn't find.

We make happiness for ourselves. It cannot be given to us although the circumstances to experience it can be prepared by others. Happiness cannot be purchased. Most certainly it cannot be put on layaway. Happiness is manufactured from life, from experience, appreciation, love, hope, time, diversity and, most often, when one shares moments of caring with others.

You need a sense of your own worthiness to find happiness. Like all valuable possessions it takes attention and practice. Jorge Luis Borges uses the Aleph to signify all there is and all you know. It is a magical lens through which you see the past and all the future, where the interrelationship of things, events and actions are comprehended. The deep place inside each of us solidifies into an Aleph through which we can see wholly, without judgment, all our experiences, all our hopes and dreams, until at last—when the center holds—happiness comes dancing in. It flies on breezes, vibrates in colors of the sunset, wafts in with the fragrance of flowers, or sings a bird's song. Happiness feasts on small things—

grandchildren, friends, witty conversation, a good book, clean windows, a sunny day or nourishing rain. Happiness and bliss grow from worthwhile tasks performed lovingly for friends and family and the self.

The capacity for joy is a talent to be nurtured. In the last decade or so, the weigh, count and measure profession has come up with a definition: happiness is a sense of subjective well-being. So? But how do you get there? One consistent finding in all my reading is that optimists are generally happier than pessimists, regardless of the actual circumstances of their lives. In part, at least, you find what you look for.

Rigidity in thoughts and actions deters us from finding or pursuing our bliss. Novelty is important. We have been taught since childhood to be consistent, to do things the "right" way, to be proud of regularity (never missed a day of work in thirty years), follow a set routine (I always wash dishes immediately). Some folks insist on finishing a book (or a project) even when the book is dumb. These and other habitual mind-sets are addictions that thwart the imagination and hold us back from full realization of our potential.

Addictions dull the mind, limit the possibilities and confine us in an intellectual and spiritual straitjacket. Perfectionists are rarely happy. The inability to accept one's own capacity realistically, striving always to be perfect, is a certain road to ulcers, broken marriages and early death. It also frequently protects the claimant from having to actually finish anything or make room for better ways to be. Keep the laziness principle in mind: *Do the most you possibly can with the least possible effort—and some style!* And let the style be the start of your bliss.

For a truly happy life, aim for frequency and duration, not intensity. Wild, joyous feelings are wonderful when they come, but not as a steady diet. Expecting peak moments all the time is unrealistic and will leave you discontented when they fail to appear.

To summarize this long journey through our lives, through literature and time, certain suggestions occur over and over. The one most often repeated, and one we know is:

Make friends and take time to be a friend. Go in search of compatible women and men, ones who share your values and interests. Reinforce each other along the way. Distribute hugs and caresses generously. Healing hands do heal.

Here are others:

Do what you like to do. Occupy yourself with fulfilling tasks. This is our time. Do what you enjoy, knowing that actions in the service of others—altruism—is basic to the survival of both individuals and the society. Relationships are strengthened by co-operation that brings us together, but torn apart by competition that separates us. No accumulation of things, money or awards will make us any better than we already are.

Take care of your body. Respect it and love it though all the changes Time imposes. Exercise, eat wisely, stay fit. Beauty comes from within, not from expensive creams and magic elixirs. Age is honorable.

Try new things and have fun. Learning is lifelong, novelty delights us. Be open to new ideas and unexpected opportunities.

Visualize the life you want and seek to create it. Depend on your intuition, your creativity and your desire to live fully, consciously with grace. Strive for conviviality. The more friendly the world around us, the more likely we are to find our bliss.

Cherish the Earth. Touch it, feel the power of the life force, protect it in whatever way you can.

Experience the highs and the lows for what they are. Both are part of the flow of life, both are inevitable. Ask yourself what an experience is teaching you, how can it make you stronger and better equipped to live your life.

Believe in yourself. Know that you are a role model for others, including our daughters and granddaughters.

Be not afraid. Choose life. Let our voices be heard in the council chambers of the mighty.

None of us will be safe at the top of the hill until the value of women's contribution to the well-being of the world is recognized.

We have the wisdom of the world available to us, accessible as never before through books, videos and computer networks. The more knowledgeable, friendly and peaceful the world we inhabit, the more likely we are to find our bliss.

The decade in which I write this book leads us to the year 2000, the beginning of a new millennium. It will be different because it *must* be different. The greedy eighties are gone, the seventies all but forgotten. The "everything goes" mind-set that characterized the sixties, and which largely excluded us from its adventures, is being replaced by a new realism characterized by a growing awareness of limits and vulnerabilities. The wasteful, ostentatious "Me Generation" is left standing stunned on clearcut hillsides, beside polluted waters, gasping fetid air.

The human family is on a renewed quest for spirituality. It will not long be content with vengeful gods existing in some distant place beyond the space probes or the range of orbiting telescopes. We will recognize the miracle of creation and the divinity around us immanent in all that is. The new humanity will cherish the holiness of life. In the foreword to the Marija Gimbutas volume, *The Language of the Goddess*, Joseph Campbell writes:

> One cannot but feel that in the appearance of this volume at just this turn of the century there is an evident relevance to the universally recognized need in our time for a general transformation of consciousness. The message here is of an actual age of harmony and peace in accord with the creative energies of nature which for a spell of some four thousand

prehistoric years anteceded the five thousand of what James Joyce has termed the "nightmare of contending tribal and national interests" from which it is now certainly time for the planet to wake.

Society has relied too long on machines and impersonal techniques. Human life requires compassion and love to make it better; so does the planet. Survival calls for a shared commitment to life in the hearts and minds of us all. Once we recognize the holiness and grandeur of our planet we will care enough to preserve it.

We will unlock the door to our personal future with keys of imagination, and with the sure knowledge that we each depend on the seamless web of life woven about our planet's fiery core. Where one sparrow falls, or one person falters, the web is rent. We ageful women must care for and love one another for our own well-being. The transcendent quality of higher consciousness is that when we reach it, we realize that what is good for us is good for everyone else. Begin to live each day as you will wish to live when the new millennium comes and the world will live as one. We will know what to do because we are old and smart!

The final step toward the full realization of the self is to take charge of our lives. It is our time. Think hard and deep about what you want the rest of your life to mean to you, what you want to achieve. Look inward to your Higher Self. List your heart's desires, your bliss. Make your plan joyfully and complete. Anything you want or wish to become will be possible in the life plan you create for yourself. Bring it into some tangible form that is available for reference whenever it seems you are slipping into old, unsatisfying patterns. This is the first day of the rest of our lives, and we are designing our existence for what time we are on this Earth. Fill it with Light. We women of years and wisdom must help in the search for loving myths, honor them, perhaps not because we want new myths but because we must find them. Our species survival requires it. The old ways of thinking are not adequate.

We have done our world much service. Throughout our lives we have prepared happiness for those who have depended on us. It is now time to include *our* heart's desires in the picture. Thank you, Age Mates, for coming with me on this journey of discovery. My life has been enriched by the task. May yours be also. Until we meet again, Blessed Be.

Let us end our journey here with the words of this brilliant document as enlightened guidance.

A Declaration of Interdependence

When in the Course of Human Events, it becomes necessary to create a new bond among the peoples of the earth, connecting each to the other, undertaking equal responsibilities under the laws of nature, a decent respect for the welfare of humankind and all life on earth requires us to Declare our Interdependence.

We recognize that humankind has not woven the web of life; we are but one thread within it. Whatever we do to the web, we do to ourselves. Whatever befalls the earth befalls also the family of the earth.

We are concerned about the wounds and bleeding sores on the naked body of the earth: the famine; the poverty; the children born into hunger and disease; the destruction of forests and fertile lands: the chemical and nuclear accidents; the wars and deaths in so many parts of the world.

It is our belief that man's dominion over nature parallels the subjugation of women in many societies, denying them sovereignty over their lives and bodies. Until all societies truly value women and the environment, their joint degradation will continue.

Women's views on economic justice, human rights, reproduction and the achievement of peace must be heard at local, national and international forums, wherever policies are made that could affect the future of life on earth. Partnership among all peoples is essential for the survival of the planet.

If we are to have a common future, we must commit ourselves to preserve the natural wealth of our earth for future generations. *As women* we accept our responsibility and declare our intention to:

- Link with others—young and old, women and men, people of all races, religions, cultures and political beliefs—in a common concern for global survival;
- Be aware in our private, public and working lives of actions we can take to safeguard our food, fresh water, clean air and quality of life;
- Make women's collective experiences and value judgments equal to the experiences and value judgments of men when policies are made that affect our future and future generations;
- Expose the connections between environmental degradation, greed, uncontrolled militarism and technology devoid of human values. Insist that human and ecological values take absolute precedence when decisions are made in national affairs;
- Change government, economic and social policies to protect the well-being of the most vulnerable among us and to end poverty and inequality;
- Work to dismantle nuclear and conventional weapons, build trust among peoples and nations, and use all available international institutions and networks to achieve common security for the family of earth.

We also declare that, whenever and wherever people meet to decide the fate of the planet, it is our intention to participate on an equal footing, with full and fair representation, equivalent to our number and kind on earth.
—Drawn from the words and philosophies of the drafters of the US Declaration of Independence (July 4, 1776); Chief Seattle to President Franklin Pierce (1855); Wangari Maathai, founder, Green Belt Movement, and Chair, National Council of Women of Kenya (1988); Women's Foreign Policy Council; The World Commission on Environment and Development (1987); Spiritual and Parliamentary Leaders Global Survival Conference, Oxford (1988) and circulated by the Movement for Ecofeminism.

Acknowledgments

Thanks are owed to many women and men, among them Seymour Trieger, partner, friend and computer consultant who suggested that I write about my life experiences under the general topic of women and aging. He even applied to Canada Council for the grant that permitted me time to research the mysteries of aging and set me on an entirely new career.

It has been my great pleasure to work with my editor, Mary Schendlinger, whose understanding is enhanced by the breadth and depth of her knowledge.

My sincere thanks to Gert Beadle, Betty Jardine, Mildred Tremblay and Pat Wheatley—Age Mates who shared their creative works and allowed me to use them. Thanks also to Howard Jerome who, with Jean Houston, wrote and performed "You Are More." Special good wishes are sent to Shakti Gawain whose valuable suggestions in *Creative Visualization* opened a path of personal discovery. Jonald Dumont introduced me to the work of Starhawk to reveal an entirely new way of thinking about women in history.

I'm indebted to the women of power and vision who have carried us this far toward equality and dignity. I am inspired by the reservoirs of information now gathering through the work of philosophers, anthropologists, scholars of many disciplines and

315

women of good purpose, who slowly chip away at the wall of ignorance that obscures women's contribution to the work of the world. At last, when new ways of knowing are urgently needed, women are beginning to speak out. Our stories are being variously told by artists and craftspersons, musicians, performers and writers. Listen well.

I urge you to tell *your* story by whatever creative means are at your disposal. Place your truth and common sense on the altar of the Mother goddess to protect it from Mammon. Turn toward values and matters of worth that you want to happen. We are all getting older *and* smarter, and the world needs to hear from us.

Sources of Interest

Adler, Margot. *Drawing Down the Moon*. Boston: Beacon Press, 1986.

Atwood, Margaret E. *The Handmaid's Tale*. Toronto: McClelland and Stewart, 1985.

Balboa, Deena and David. *Walk for Life: the Lifetime Walking Program for a Healthy Body and Mind*. New York: Perigee Books, 1990.

Benedict, Ruth. *Patterns of Culture*. Boston: Houghton Mifflin, 1961.

Benson, Herbert. *The Relaxation Response*. New York: W.F. Morrow & Co., 1976.

_____, and William Proctor. *Your Maximum Mind*. New York: Times Books, 1987.

Beresford-Howe, Constance. *The Book of Eve*. Toronto: Macmillan, 1973.

Berman, Morris. *The Reenchantment of the World*. Ithaca NY: Cornell University Press, 1981.

Berner, Mark, and Gerald Rotenberg, eds. *Guide to Prescription and Over the Counter Drugs*. Montreal: Canadian Medical Association and Readers Digest Association, 1990.

Bolles, Richard Nelson. *What Color is Your Parachute?* Berkeley: Ten Speed Press, 1972. (See latest edition).

Boston Women's Health Collective. *Our Bodies, Ourselves: A Book By and For Women*. New York: Simon and Schuster, 1976.

_____. *The New Our Bodies, Ourselves*. New York: Touchstone Press, 1992.

_____. Doress, Paula Brown and Diana Laskin Siegal, eds. *Ourselves, Growing Older: Women Aging with Knowledge and Power*. New York: Simon and Schuster, 1987.

Bricklin, Mark, Robert Bendiner, eds. *Positive Living and Health: The Complete Guide to Brain/Body Healing and Mental Empowerment*. Emmaus PA: Rodale Press, 1990.

Brothers, Joyce. *Widowed*. New York: Ballantine Press, 1992.

Brownmiller, Susan. *Femininity*. New York: Fawcett Columbine, 1984.

Brundtland, Gro Harlem, Chair. The World Commission on Environment and Development. *Our Common Future*. New York: Oxford University Press, 1987.

Callenbach, Ernest. *Ecotopia*. New York: Bantam Books, 1975.

Campbell, Joseph. *The Masks of God: Creative Mythology*. New York: Viking Penguin, 1968.

_____. *The Hero with a Thousand Faces*. Princeton: Princeton University Press, 1949.

_____. *Primitive Mythology*. New York: Viking, 1959.

_____. *The Power of Myth*. New York: Doubleday, 1988.

Chopra, Deepak. *Ageless Body, Timeless Mind: The Quantum Alternative to Growing Old*. New York: Harmony Books (Crown), 1993.

Cohen, Leah. *Small Expectations: Society's Betrayal of Older Women*. Toronto: McClelland and Stewart Ltd., 1984.

Cousins, Norman. *Anatomy of an Illness: Reflections on Healing and Regeneration*. New York: Norton, 1979.

Daly, Mary. *Gyn/Ecology: The Metaethics of Radical Feminism*. Boston: Beacon Press, 1978.

De Beauvoir, Simone. *The Coming of Age*. New York: Putnam, 1972.

_____. *The Second Sex*. New York: Alfred A. Knopf, 1953.

De Ropp, Robert S. *Sex Energy. The Sexual Force in Man and Animals*. New York: Dell, 1969.

Doress, Paula Brown and Diana Laskin Siegal, eds. *Ourselves, Growing Older: Women Aging with Knowledge and Power*. New York: Simon and Schuster, 1987.

Dychtwald, Ken and Joe Flower. *Age Wave: the Challenges and Opportunities of an Aging North America*. Los Angeles: J.P. Tarcher, Inc., 1988.

Edwards, Betty. *Drawing on the Artist Within*. New York: Simon and Schuster, 1986.

_____. *Drawing on the Right Side of the Brain*. Los Angeles: J.P. Tarcher, 1979.

Ehrenreich, Barbara and English, Deirdre. *Witches, Midwives and Nurses: A History of Women Healers*. New York: The Feminist Press, 1973.

Eisler, Riane. *The Chalice and the Blade: Our History, Our Future*. New York: Harper & Row, 1988.

Elgin, Duane. *Voluntary Simplicity: An Ecological Lifestyle that Promotes Personal and Social Renewal*. New York: Bantam Books, 1982.

Ferguson, Marilyn. *The Aquarian Conspiracy, Personal and Social Transformation in the 1980's*. Los Angeles: J.P. Tarcher, 1980.

Frazer, Sir James G. *The Golden Bough*. New York: Macmillan, 1922.

French, Marilyn. *Beyond Power: On Women, Men, and Morals*. New York: Ballantine Books, 1985.

Friedan, Betty. "Television and the Feminine Mystique." *TV Guide*, Vol. 12, No. 5, February 1964.

_____. *The Feminine Mystique*. New York: Dell, 1963.

_____. *The Second Stage*. New York: Simon and Schuster, 1981.

_____. *The Fountain of Age*. New York: Simon and Schuster, 1993.

Garcia, Gabriel Marquez. *Love in the Time of Cholera*. New York: Alfred A. Knopf, 1988.

Gawain, Shakti. *Creative Visualization*. Mill Valley CA: Whatever Publishing, Inc. 1978.

Gimbutas, Marija. *The Language of the Goddess: Unearthing the Hidden Symbols of Western Civilization*. New York: HarperCollins, 1991

Greer, Germaine. *Sex and Destiny: The Politics of Human Fertility*. New York: Harper and Row Publishers, 1984.

Griscom. Chris. *Ecstasy is a New Frequency*. New York: Simon and Schuster, 1987.

Hen Co-op Staff. *Growing Old Disgracefully: New Ideas For Getting the Most Out of Life*. Freedom CA: The Crossing Press, 1994.

Henderson, Hazel. *The Politics of the Solar Age: Alternatives to Economics*. Indianapolis IN: Knowledge Systems Inc., 1988.

Hilliard, Marion. *A Women Doctor Looks at Life and Love*. Garden City NY: Doubleday, 1956.

Hoopes, Ned E., ed. *Who Am I? Essays on the Alienated*. New York: Dell, 1969.

Houston, Jean and Howard Jerome Gomberg. *You Are More: Songs of the Possible Human*. Audiocassette. Portland: The Greater Spiral, Oregon, 1983.

_____. *The Possible Human*. Los Angeles: J.P. Tarcher, 1982.

_____. *Life Force: The Psycho-Historical Recovery Of The Self*. New York: Dell, 1980.

Huxley, Aldous. *The Doors of Perception*. New York: Harper & Row, 1963.

Illich, Ivan. *Limits to Medicine: Medical Nemesis: the Expropriation of Health*. New York: Penguin, 1977.

Jampolsky, Gerald G. *Good-Bye to Guilt: Releasing Fear Through Forgiveness*. New York: Bantam Books, 1985.

Johnson, Sonia. *Going Out of Our Minds: the Metaphysics of Liberation*. Freedom CA: Crossing Press, 1987.

Kalweit, Holger. *Dreamtime and Inner Space*. Boston: Shambhala Publications, 1988.

Kapleau, Philip, ed. *Three Pillars of Zen: Teaching, Practice and Enlightenment*. Boston: Beacon Press 1967.

Keyes, Ken, Jr. *Handbook to Higher Consciousness*. Coos Bay OR: Living Love Publications, 1986.

Kübler-Ross, Elisabeth. *On Death and Dying*. New York: Macmillan, 1969.

_____. *Death: The Final Stage of Growth*. Englewood Cliffs NJ: Prentice-Hall, 1975.

Kuhn, Maggie. "The Gray Panthers: Networking for New Community." *Dromenon* (New York NY), Vol. II, No. 1, June 1979.

Lappé, Frances Moore. *Diet for a Small Planet*. New York: Ballantine Books, 1991. (References are to 1971 edition).

Larousse Encyclopedia of Mythology. London: Hamlyn Publishing Group, 1968.

Le Shan, ed. *It's Better to Be Over the Hill Than Under It: Thoughts on Life Over Sixty*. New York: Newmarket Press, 1990.

_____. *The Wonderful Crisis of Middle Age*. New York: Warner Books, 1973.

Marian, John J. "Health Care Rights: a Position Paper." Saskatoon SK: Association of Mental Health, 1975.

_____. *Needless Surgery*. Saskatoon SK: Association on Human Rights, 1976.

Masters, Robert, and Jean Houston. *Mind Games: The Guide to Inner Space*. New York: Dell, 1972.

Millett, Kate. *Sexual Politics*. New York: Avon Books (Doubleday), 1969.

Montagu, Ashley. *Growing Young*. Granby MA: Bergin & Garvey, 1981.

_____. *The Natural Superiority of Women*. New York: Macmillan, 1952.

Moody, Raymond A. *Life After Life: Investigation of a Phenomenon—Survival of Bodily Death*. New York: New Bantam/Mockingbird,1977.

Murray, Margaret. *The God of the Witches*. London: Oxford University Press, 1970.

Naisbitt, John. *Megatrends: Ten New Directions Transforming Our Lives*. New York: Warner Books, 1984.

Nickerson, Betty. *Celebrate the Sun*. Toronto: McClelland and Stewart, 1969. (US edition—New York: Lippincott, 1969.)

_____. *Chi: Letters from Biafra*. Toronto: New Press, 1971.

_____, ed. *All About Us/Nous Autres: Creative Writing, Painting, Drawing. A Book by and for Young People*. Montreal: Content Publishing Ltd. 1973.

_____, ed. *Girls Will Be Women: Femmes de Demain*. Ottawa: All About

Us/Nous Autres, 1975.

Nickerson, Michael. *Bakavi: Change the World, I Want to Stay On*. Ottawa: All About Us Books, 1977.

Nin, Anais. *In Favor of the Sensitive Man and other Essays*. New York: First Harvest (Harcourt Brace Jovanovich), 1976.

Nouwen, Henri J. M., and Walter J. Gaffney. *Aging: The Fulfillment of Life*. New York: Doubleday, 1974.

Painter, Charlotte, and Pamela Valois. *Gifts of Age*. San Francisco: Chronicle Books, 1985.

Pauling, Linus. *How to Live Longer and Feel Better*. New York: W. H. Freeman, 1986.

Pratt, Marilynn J. *God's Femininity Recognized*. Playa Del Rey CA: Golden Puer Publishing Co., 1980.

Province of British Columbia. *Choosing Wellness: An Approach to Healthy Aging*. Victoria: Ministry of Health, 1988.

Rhodes, Ann. *Guidance and Support in Caring for the Elderly*. Montreal: Grosvenor House Publishing, 1990.

Robbins, John. *Diet for a New America*. Walpole NH: Stillpoint Publishing, 1987.

Roberts, Jane. *Seth: Dreams and Projection of Consciousness*. Walpole NH: Stillpoint Publishing, 1987.

Robin, Eugene Debs. *Matters of Life and Death: Risks vs. Benefits of Medical Care*. New York: W. H. Freeman, 1984.

Russell, J. B. *Witchcraft in the Middle Ages*. Ithaca: Cornell University Press, 1972.

Santayana, George. *The Birth of Reason and Other Essays*. New York: Columbia University Press, 1968.

Satin, Mark. *New Age Politics: Healing Self and Society*. Vancouver BC: Whitecap Books, 1978.

Satir, Virginia. *Peoplemaking*. Palo Alto CA: Science and Behavior Books, Inc. 1972.

Senter, Sylvia, Marguerite Howe and Donald A. Saco. *Women at Work. A Psychologist's Secrets to Getting Ahead in Business*. New York: Putnam, 1982.

Siegel, Bernie S. *Peace, Love and Healing: Bodymind Communication and the Path to Self-Healing: An Exploration*. New York: Harper and Row, 1989.

Silber, Sherman J. *The Male from Infancy to Old Age*. New York: Charles Scribner's Sons, 1981.

Smith, Betty. *A Tree Grows In Brooklyn*. New York: Harper, 1943.

Smith, Homer. *Man and His Gods*. Boston: Little Brown, 1952.

Spangler, David. "Economics as a Way of the Spirit." *Onearth*. Forres, Scotland:

Findhorn Foundation, 1979.

Starhawk. *Dreaming the Dark: Magic, Sex and Politics*. Boston: Beacon Press, 1982.

_____. *The Spiral Dance: A Rebirth of the Ancient Religion of the Great Goddess*. New York: Harper and Row, 1983.

Steinbeck, John. *The Grapes of Wrath*. New York: Viking, 1939.

Steinem, Gloria. *Revolution from Within: a Book of Self-Esteem*. Boston: Little, Brown, 1992.

Stone, Merlin. *When God Was a Woman*. New York: Dial Press, 1976.

Terkel, Studs. *The Great Divide: Second Thoughts on the American Dream*. New York: Avon Books, 1988.

Twain, Mark. *Letters from the Earth*. Greenwich CN.: Fawcett, 1938.

Ueland, Brenda. *If You Want to Write*. St. Paul MN: Graywolf Press, 1938.

Vande Kieft, Kathleen. *Innersource*. New York: Ballantine/New Age, 1988.

Walker, Barbara G. *The Woman's Encyclopedia of Myths and Secrets*. San Francisco: Harper & Row, 1983.

_____. *The Crone: Woman of Age, Wisdom, and Power*. San Francisco: Harper & Row, 1985.

Ward, Barbara. *The Interplay of East and West*. New York: Norton, 1962.

West, Robin L., and Jan D. Sinnot, eds. *Everyday Memory and Aging: Current Research and Methodology*. New York: Springer-Verlag, 1992.

Wilkinson, Loren, ed. *Earthkeeping: Christian Stewardship of Natural Resources*. Grand Rapids MI: W. B. Eerdmans, 1980.

Zukav, Gary. *The Dancing Wu Li Masters: An Overview of the New Physics*. New York: William Morrow, 1979.

_____. *The Seat of the Soul*. New York: Fireside (Simon and Schuster), 1989.

INDEX

abortion, 218, 224
abuse of aging women, 233, 236–38, 240–44
addictions, 227–30, 308
advertising, 30, 86, 185–90; *see also* consumerism
Affirmations of Maturity, 88–89
Age Mates, definition, 33–34
alcohol, 230
Alphabet of Time, 65
altruistic egoism, 84
Alzheimer's disease, see memory fitness
Amazing Grays, 68–69, 165–67, 203
anger, 231–33
art, 167–68

barter, 264
Beadle, Gert, 247–48
beauty, 28, 73–88, 309
Bedtime Story, 247–48
birth control, 216–19, 223–24
birthdays, 67–72
bladder control, 80–81
body image, 73–88, 193
Brothers, Joyce, 284–85

caesarean section, 145
Campbell, Joseph, 306, 310–11

cancer, 81–82, 120, 144–45
caring for aged parents, 239–40
Chicago, Judy, 167–68
childhood, 40–42
child raising, *see* work
Christianity, 112–13, 234
circle, women's, 93–98
civil rights movement, 61–62
clothes, 55–56, 263–64
Cold War, 60–62
community, 33–37, 68–69, 82, 85, 91–97, 164–65, 169–71, 173–74, 240, 245–46, 309
consumerism, 28, 55–56, 185–90, 252; *see also* advertising
creative visualization, 82, 126–29
Croning Party, 68
culture-giving, 103–110
cyprine (vaginal fluid), 225–26

dance, 174–77
Davis, Adele, 185
day trips, 262
DBL (Depression, Boredom, Loneliness), 199–200, 272–88
death, 152, 289–304; *see also* hospices, Near Death Experience
depression, 38–39, 57–58, 272–88

Depression, Boredom, Loneliness (DBL), 199–200, 272–88
Depression, 1930s, 26, 42–45, 220
diet, 79, 184–94, 198, 199, 261
Dinner Party, The, 167–68
"Dishing It Up to Mrs. Corbeau," 58–59
divorce, 221–22, 286–87; *see also* relationships
doctors, *see* medical profession
drinking, 230
drugs, prescription, 63, 125, 142, 147–50, 198–99, 261, 277
dyspimea, 277; *see also* depression

Earth, celebration ritual, 93–98
Earth, preservation of, 29, 31–32, 45, 69, 91–98, 107–108, 135–36, 171, 311, 312–14
empty nest syndrome, 38; *see also* depression
environmental issues, *see* Earth
euthanasia, *see* right to die
exercise, 86, 178–83, 309

families, 245–46
Feminine Mystique, The, 38–39, 57–58
financial planning, *see* money
food, *see* diet
food gathering, *see* work
food supply, 184–94, 261
Friedan, Betty, 38–39, 57–58
friends, *see* community

gardening, 164–65, 182, 191–92
geriatrics, 139, 152
gerontology, 139
goddesses and gods, *see* spirituality
grief, 272–88

healing mind, 77, 81, 83, 111–36, 306–207
health, alternative therapies, 142–43, 158–77, 231–33; and art, 167–68; and being centered, 76; and body image, 73–88; and dance, 174–77; definition, 156; diet, 186–94; drinking, 230; exercise, 178–83; gardening, 164–65; hobbies,

168–69; laughter, 158–60; music, 172–74; and pets, 161–64; and play, 165–67; sexually transmitted diseases, 215, 217; smoking, 227–30; studies on healthy older women, 77–78; tears, 171–72; toys, 168–69; volunteering, 169–71; World Health Organization definition, 115; *see also* community, healing mind, medical profession, spirituality
heart disease, 120
historical record, women in, 24–26, 38–66
hobbies, 168–69
homemaking, *see* work
hormone therapy, 77–78
hospices, 152, 299
hospitals, 146
House Rules for Husbands, 243–44
housing, 258–61
Howe, Julia Ward, 106
husband, tyrant, 240–45
hysterectomy, 144–45

Ibo Age Mates, 34
immigrants to North America, 41
incontinence, 80–81
intuition, 280–83
isometrics, 179

Kegel maneuver, 80

language, 33–34
laughter, 159, 273–74
Laziness Principle, 250
LETS (Local Employment Trading System), 264
Letter to My Doctor, 152–54
life-based pursuits, 28
light deprivation, 278–79
lobbying, 253–55
Local Employment Trading System (LETS), 264
loneliness, 35, 82

marriage, *see* relationships
Maturity, Affirmations of, 88–89
MBO (Mind, Body, Others), 183

medical profession, 137–57; choosing a doctor, 154–56; geriatrics, 139, 152; gerontology, 139; hospitals, 146; Letter to My Doctor, 152–54; and male patients, 138; patients' rights, 150–54; second opinions, 144–47; self-regulation, 147; and sexuality, 207–208; specialists, 140–41; surgery, 144–47; technology, 140–41; women medical students, 139–40; *see also* drugs
medicine, natural, 142
medicine wheel, 93–98
meditation, 129–34
memory fitness, 195–205
menopause, 69, 77–78, 208
Mind, Body, Others (MBO), 183
money, 28–29, 249–71; barter, 264; clothes, 263–64; day trips, 262; economic discrimination against women, 253–54; economic power of seniors, 252; food, 261; housing, 258–61; 100 Things to Do That Don't Cost Any Money, 270–71; seniors' discounts, 21; travel, 262; voluntary simplicity, 267–68; volunteering, 262; wills, 265–67; *see also* consumerism, Depression, pensions
Mother's Day Proclamation, 105–106
music, 172–74

NAB (Negativity, Anger and Bitterness), 125–26
Near Death Experience, 290–96
Negativity, Anger and Bitterness (NAB), 125–26
networking, *see* community
"New Age," 89–98; *see also* spirituality
nutrition, *see* diet

100 Things to Do That Don't Cost Any Money, 270–71
Ozymandias, 103–104

patients' rights, 150–54
Pauling, Linus, 143–44
peacemaking, 53–54, 60–61, 62–63, 103–110, 216
pension, 20, 59, 250, 252–53, 255–56
Perfect Retired Couple, 244
pets, 161–64
PhT (Putting Hubby Through), 59
physical changes, 73–88, 225–26
pineal gland, 126, 279–80
play, 165–67
poverty, 102, 250, 255–56
praying, 84–85
prescriptions, *see* drugs
psychosomatic illness, *see* healing mind
purple, 36–37

rape, 237–38
recycling, 26, 50–51; *see also* Earth
relationships, 81–82, 240–46; *see also* sexuality
relaxation response, 130
religion, *see* spirituality
retirement, 242–44
rights, patients', 150–54
right to die, 297–300
Rodriguez, Sue, 297–98
Roosevelt, Franklin D., 44–45
Ross, Betsy, 24

second opinion, medical, 144–47
Secord, Laura, 24
Selye, Hans, 84
senility, definition, 197–98
seniors' centers, 35–36
seniors' discounts, 21, 261–62
sexuality, 206–226; and body image, 73–88
sexually transmitted diseases, 215, 217, 226
sexual revolution, 1960s, 64, 215–16, 220–21
Siegel, Bernie, 119–20
smoking, 227–30
specialists, 140–41
spirituality, 89–98, 111–13, 202–203, 267–69, 280–83, 289–304, 305–314; *see also* healing mind, meditation, visualization

stretching, 179
Sundowner's syndrome, 278–79
support, *see* community
surgery, 144–47

Tai Chi, 181
tax credits, 20
tears, 171–72
television, 262–63
thrivsil, 156–57
toys, 168–69
transcendental meditation, 129–34
travel, 262
Tremblay, Mildred, 204–205

vaginal fluid (cyprine), 225–26
Venus of Willendorf, 73
Vietnam war, 63
violence, 233–39, 303; *see also* peacemaking, war
visualization, 82, 126–29, 309
Voice of Women, 62
voluntary simplicity, 267–68
volunteering, 169–71, 262

walking, 180–81

war, 24, 45–46, 236, 303–304; celebrations, 303; Vietnam, 63; World War One, 45–46; World War Two, 48–55, 219–20; *see also* peacemaking
wellness, *see* health
Wheatley, Patience, 58–59
widowhood, 272–88
wills, 265–67
witch hunts, 234–35
"Woman in the Mirror, The," 83
women in historical record, 24–26, 38–66
women's circle, 93–98
women's liberation movement, 63, 215–16
women's suffrage, 25, 44
work, 23–24, 59–60, 64; and preservation of Earth, 107–108; child raising, 55–66, 99–110; during World War Two, 50–55; food gathering, 102, 184; homemaking, 55–66, 99–110; in 1920s and 1930s, 39–40; and quality of society, 102–103; re-entering the workforce, 256–57
writing, 231

yoga, 181–82
"You Are More," 121–23